THE
CULINARY
PHARMACY

"*The Culinary Pharmacy* is not just a book on healthy eating; it is a recipe for living a healthy life. Within the pages of this book are recipes and mindfulness techniques woven together with holistic dietary practices from around the world. Having worked with Lisa personally on my path to health and recommended Lisa's services to many of my clients, I am thrilled to see Lisa's knowledge of food as medicine shared in these pages!"

SALICROW, PSYCHIC MEDIUM AND AUTHOR OF
THE PATH OF ELEMENTAL WITCHCRAFT AND
SPIRIT SPEAKER: A MEDIUM'S GUIDE TO DEATH AND DYING

THE
CULINARY
PHARMACY

Intuitive Eating,
Ancestral Healing,
and Your
Personal Nutrition Plan

LISA MASÉ

Healing Arts Press
Rochester, Vermont

Healing Arts Press
One Park Street
Rochester, Vermont 05767
www.HealingArtsPress.com

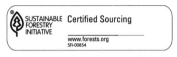

Text stock is SFI certified

Healing Arts Press is a division of Inner Traditions International

The author's poems "The Songs Become My Home" (see chapter 1), "Bread Ghazal" (see chapter 4), "Origins" (see chapter 5), and "Papi Mi Ha Insegnato" (see chapter 9) were originally published in her book *I Won't Be/long Here* by Kelsay Books in American Fork, Utah, in 2021.

Note to the reader: *This book is intended as an informational guide. The remedies, approaches, and techniques described herein are meant to supplement, and not to be a substitute for, professional medical care or treatment. They should not be used to treat a serious ailment without prior consultation with a qualified health care professional.*

Cataloging-in-Publication Data for this title is available from the Library of Congress

ISBN 978-1-64411-864-1 (print)
ISBN 978-1-64411-865-8 (ebook)

Printed and bound in the United States by Lake Book Manufacturing, LLC
The text stock is SFI certified. The Sustainable Forestry Initiative® program promotes sustainable forest management.

10 9 8 7 6 5 4 3 2 1

Text design and layout by Kenleigh Manseau
This book was typeset in Garamond Premier Pro with Haboro Contrast and Forma DJR Micro used as display typefaces

To send correspondence to the author of this book, mail a first-class letter to the author c/o Inner Traditions • Bear & Company, One Park Street, Rochester, VT 05767, and we will forward the communication, or contact the author directly at **harmonized-living.com**.

Contents

Foreword

By Rosemary Gladstar

You're in for a delightful treat. Healthy living not only feels great but tastes fabulous as well! Lisa Masé, author of *The Culinary Pharmacy,* is a chef, herbalist, and nutritionist, and she has a tremendous amount to share with us. Lisa is a beloved member of a loosely knit community of herbalists and healers, chefs, gardeners, artists, musicians, and craftspeople who live in the central Vermont area. I first met Lisa shortly after she moved to Vermont. She was a vibrant, energetic young woman—before she became desperately ill with a chronic life-threatening disease. I knew her during those years when she bravely struggled to find answers for a rare and devastating illness, though little to no information about her disease seemed forthcoming. I knew her when she was painfully thin and exhausted a great deal of the time, seeming to have little energy to carry on. And I witnessed her valiant and determined effort to find her way back to health and radiant well-being. This is Lisa's story . . . but hers is far more than a compelling and inspiring personal journey of health and healing. Lisa is also incredibly well informed on matters of wellness, working from a base of knowledge earned through her own personal experiences, her work as a professional health and nutritional consultant, and her ongoing research and studies. This compilation of knowledge, wisdom, and practical experience is what she so readily and generously shares in the pages of *The Culinary Pharmacy.*

The wisdom woven into these pages can help each of us achieve a healthier, more radiant life. In *The Culinary Pharmacy,* we learn about constitutional types, metagenomics, enterotypes, bacterial ecosystems, intuitive eating, and the importance of food sovereignty, as well as a variety of healing modalities and compatible but different approaches to healing. While Lisa provides abundant resources for further research, she does an excellent job of distilling the information into meaningful bite-size portions that don't overwhelm. Her approach, which I appreciate fully, is to make this information not only understandable and approachable but also, and more importantly, doable. I can actually take the steps she encourages and recommends. If I can take these steps, if she could, then we all can. That in itself is quite an accomplishment, because illness, especially chronic long-term illness, can be overwhelming not only to the patient but to the patient's family and caregivers. It is often hard to know where to start, who to believe, what to do. But as Lisa wisely states, "We do not strive for perfection; we aim for progress." She encourages us to begin with small steps to shift habits and then instructs us how to put into practice those things that will make a positive difference in our lives.

While *The Culinary Pharmacy* is overflowing with practical information, simple practices, and manageable steps we can take to improve our health and well-being, it is also richly embellished with stories of the land, of food, of family and community. Lisa doesn't separate the health of an individual from the health of the land and community. Instead, she shows us, these are woven intricately together: healthy land, healthy community, healthier individuals. She herself learned about these ideas as a child growing up in a small mountain village in northern Italy. These early lessons informed and impacted Lisa's childhood, her personal healing journey, and later her healing work with others. Many of the teachings Lisa brings to the table were lessons learned from her Italian grandmother, Nonna Dina, and her wise father, who took his young children into the forest to teach them about the healing plants and wild mushrooms that grew there. From these early experiences Lisa learned that "the healing power of food comes both from what we eat and how we eat it. . . . The sacred act of preparing and savoring food is the foundation for who we are."

Given her emphasis on food and nutrition as a primary cornerstone of healing and healthy living, it's only natural that Lisa would share many of her favorite recipes, and, most specifically, the recipes that helped her heal. However, unlike many traditional cookbooks, these recipes aren't organized into separate chapters according to appetizers, soups, main dishes, and such. Instead, they are woven into Lisa's teachings and stories. Food is what heals, and where our food comes from and how it's prepared and savored all matter. Throughout *The Culinary Pharmacy*, Lisa kindly and wisely directs us to the kitchen, to food, and to the wise intelligence of our enteric brain, the gut. And she does so with such deliciousness. I've tried many of Lisa's recipes and can vouch for how pleasurable, satisfying, and easy "healthy eating" can be!

With determination, help, and guidance, Lisa did find her way back to health. Lisa is a parent of two small children, a partner, and a professional health consultant who lives a richly full and active life. When our paths cross, as they do from time to time, I once again see that vibrant healthy woman I first met so many years ago, though she's been graced with the wisdom and maturity that comes only with life's experiences. No one would ever want or wish illness on another, but using each life lesson that comes to us as an opportunity to grow and, furthermore, to help others on their journey, is one of the arts of living well. As Lisa so aptly says, "Seeing illness as a blessing has allowed me to learn from it and hold space for others to learn as well." This book is Lisa's gift of wellness to us; it is her "holding space for others to learn." It is filled with simple earth-based wisdom about how to live fuller, more balanced, and vibrant lives through the food choices we make and the habits we cultivate.

As Lisa says, "The more we take charge of how we want to relate to our food, our days, and our world, the more we become empowered to heal ourselves through the daily activities that shape our world." Thank you, Lisa, for showing the way.

ROSEMARY GLADSTAR
HERBALIST AND AUTHOR
FROM HER HOME ON MISTY BAY, VERMONT

Rosemary Gladstar is internationally renowned in the field of modern herbalism for her technical knowledge and stewardship in the global herbalist community. She has been learning, teaching, and writing about herbs for over forty years and is the author of eleven books. Her works include *Medicinal Herbs: A Beginner's Guide, Herbal Healing for Women, Rosemary Gladstar's Herbal Recipes for Vibrant Health,* and *The Science and Art of Herbalism.* She also created an in-depth home-study course and is a founder and president of United Plant Savers and founder and past director of the International Herb Symposium.

Preface
Honoring Origins and Intuition

I am a white, colonist, Italian American, emigrated, gender-fluid human and prefer they or she pronouns. I walk in the realms of holistic nutrition, folk herbalism, ritual, parenting, cooking, activism, nature diving, translation, music, and poetry. I have the privilege of being a child, sibling, partner, parent, friend, accomplice, and community member. I steward unceded Abenaki land in Indokina, whose colonized name is Vermont, or the Green Mountains. I was raised near the Dolomite Mountains and the Adriatic Sea, eating the mushrooms and berries I wildcrafted with my grandmother and the food we made from scratch with our extended family. In the story of my upbringing, food is the connection between people, place, and spirit. Without nourishment, we would not live. Without the wisdom traditions centered around food, we would not thrive. I offer my gratitude to all who raised me, people and plants alike. I am deeply indebted to all the teachers, healers, and loved ones who hold me, witness me, and support me as I experience illness and restore balance, time and again. Your names are many, and I honor you with my whole being.

As I write this book, we are in an ongoing crisis of understanding how to honor all the ways to be a human being. This honoring requires a deep, hard look into our ancestry and a continued evolution of consciousness toward collective liberation. We are three years into a global pandemic. Coronavirus bloomed a hundred years after the last great global pandemic, sparked by influenza. I believe the next pandemic will come sooner than the last one. How has the world's response to this virus been shaped by the media? How has fear affected our choices? I ask these questions because they pertain both to global health and to personal wellness. In our journey to restore and maintain health, we all must find ways to separate ourselves from external, unconscious influences so we may trust intuition once again.

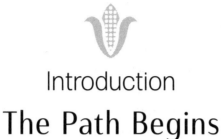

Introduction
The Path Begins

Whether intentionally or not, my parents primed my brother and me to be academics. Their careers were focused on scientific translation and geotechnics. My mom translated archaeological books of great fame, and my dad was the head of the geology department at the University of Ferrara in Italy. They praised us for being well-rounded in visual arts, poetry, fencing, soccer, and tennis. However, our highest achievements were always school-related. Since I spoke five languages by the age of ten, they thought I would graduate from college and forge a career working as a simultaneous translator.

I tried to follow the path that had been set out for me. After college, I applied to the highest-level translation agencies, but when they offered me positions, I didn't accept. Instead, I went to Indonesia. I had spent six months there as a college student, and in that time, I learned more than I ever had in any school. I found something meaningful, something transformative, in that traditional way of life.

Having felt that spark of connection to ancient ways of being, it made sense, later, after having spent years suffering from chronic intestinal parasites, to turn to traditional medicine for relief. Only after I let go of the conventional medical approach of eradicating infection with antibiotics did I start to truly appreciate the difference between curing symptoms and healing root causes. I discovered my own body as my deepest source of learning, and my disease became my teacher. Through this process, I learned to befriend my body and to create rituals that felt supportive to my physical healing. Studying traditional healing modalities such as Ayurveda and Chinese medicine helped me understand how my body was affected by my illness and recognize the importance of personalized nutrition based on both genetics (constitution) and epigenetics (conditions). I returned to the practices with which my family raised me, which centered around daily life, attention to wellness, and eating in harmony with nature.

By taking charge of my own healing process, I was able to know my body, mind, and spirit on a deeper level so that, when things became imbalanced once again, I could feel confident in my capacity to work in partnership with my whole being to heal myself. Today, I honor the blessing of illness, because it has culminated in this opportunity to share the gifts I have gained through embracing disharmony to create harmony.

What I've learned is this: the only thing we can trust is that life is ever changing. Health is defined by our ability to move at the pace of change. I honor the sacred truth of story and its capacity to constantly change, to harmonize with the moment. Each one of us has stories that inform our lives. From our own life experience to those handed down from our ancestors, there is hope and heartache, injury and repair. My story is no different than yours. We are all unique threads that are woven together, drops of water riding the waves. By looking more closely at the way humans have practiced the art of nourishment for centuries, we begin to realize that we are all one. Our practices are informed by nature, the great unifier to which we all belong.

> *At some point, I realized food was a tool for bringing people together, for telling stories about people, for telling stories about culture.*
>
> SAMIN NOSRAT

Please use this book as a vehicle for self-empowerment. It is written in the spirit of inclusion and compassion and contains stories, recipes, poetry, activism, and ideas for finding personal wellness. Know that I am on the healing path with you, learning through my body each time I encounter a new challenge and making mistakes along the way. We must all sacrifice in this lifetime. The knowledge gained through sacrifice becomes sacred, a teaching to revere in the temple of inner knowing. Consider this book as a mirror that helps you understand and embrace yourself, your loved ones, and those who came before you for the benefit of all beings. I honor your journey, recognize the challenge and promise of ancestral healing, and offer you gratitude for taking the time to consider these words and their resonance in your own life.

The Roots of Food as Medicine

Ancestral and Individual Origins

Over many years, I found that if I could relate to food with warmhearted compassion, eventually I could learn to treat people with love and respect, and I could touch my own wounds with tenderness.

EDWARD ESPE BROWN

The sense of timelessness is what first drew me to cooking. I remember standing on a chair at my grandmother's stove, tending a pot of freshly picked apricots. I could have been stirring for minutes or hours. It didn't matter. I watched, enraptured, as the sweet-tart fruit bubbled into jam. This summer ritual of making preserves has followed me in my travels. After I moved to my mom's hometown, Kansas City, as a pre-teen, I continued to find ways to cook traditional foods. I would invite new friends over for homemade pasta or crostata, an Italian fruit pie, which I always nostalgically filled with apricot jam.

Both as a teen and in my early twenties, I had the great fortune of spending time in Santa Fe, New Mexico, a place where food—especially corn and indigenous red and green chile—is considered sacred. After college I lived in an old, two-story adobe house with a fireplace and views of the Sangre de Cristo Mountains. An apricot tree reigned in our small courtyard. Its branches drooped heavy with fruit each July. I made so many jars of the delectable amber spread one summer that we gifted some to each of our neighbors.

It may have taken me three days to complete the canning project, but I did not care. I was transported by the love of working in partnership with nature in order to create an offering for others to enjoy. Not only does food bridge personal experiences, it also connects people. We share food to remember what's most vital, which is our connection to the earth. We come from and return to the same earth in which our food grows.

As author Barbara Kingsolver so aptly put it, "living takes life." We are a small part of the eternal cycle of death, rebirth, and everything in between. A song of the Yoruba tribe, "Hunger," hails, "There is no god like one's stomach. / We must sacrifice to it every day." The word *hunger* is so ancient that it appears to have co-arisen in Anatolia, the Black Sea steppes, and the Indian subcontinent centuries ago—and the original form of this word sounds much like the modern English version. Hunger drives development. First, a child cries as it takes a breath, its first source of nourishment. Then, it cries for food. Once human beings learn how to feed themselves, they learn how to interact with their environment, which changes according to season and location.

I remember the first time I watched, mystified, as my uncle fried zucchini slices on a scorching dolomitic limestone boulder under which he had built a fire. We were spending one of our many summers in the high mountains where Italy meets Austria, wandering the woods in search of mushrooms and returning to a farmhouse with red-checkered curtains, a wood cookstove, candles for nighttime light, and a hand pump for well water.

My uncle, preparing the zucchini, was unhurried, tending the fire, slicing the zucchini, and talking as he worked. The important part of the process was not how long it took but the alchemy of fire and the flavor imparted by the calcium-rich stone. After many rounds of vegetables had cooked and we had slowly feasted on them, my uncle or father would pull a pot out of the fire, and we would enjoy a mushroom and tomato stew called goulash. These vegetable-intensive feasts would be peppered with slices of hardtack rye bread, chunks of Fontina cheese, and thin rounds of summer sausage that we had hiked up in backpacks from our hometown of Bressanone.

This Austrian-Italian town where my relatives still live is just as settled in its Tyrolean ways as the majestic mountains that stood here since before human settlement. Many of the elders in this area do not quite grasp the concept of email. They prefer landlines to cell phones. During a visit with our Italian family, my father and I took a morning drive to Maso Pineto, an old farmhouse-turned-rest-stop for hikers. We passed many local dairy farmers waiting by the narrow, twisting roads for the daily milk pickup.

Instead of building technological infrastructure like cell phone towers, this region has advanced through agricultural product subsidies, which include twenty-gallon stainless-steel containers with wheels for temporary milk storage and large milk trucks to visit each village and collect the precious liquid. I was struck by the intersection of traditional methods and modern conveniences—by the wrinkled old men and women with their blue aprons, felted hats, and wool coats, patiently standing next to brand-new stainless-steel milk transport containers. Instead of looking to the outside world to define its standards, this region stands firm in valuing the land itself as its most precious asset.

Though this mindset framed the traditions in which I was raised, I lost touch with this simple way of life. Assimilation is a powerful force. I came to Kansas City for eighth grade because my mother, a native, needed to care for her aging parents. I saw that people here drove instead of walking, did not grow vegetables, and ate primarily brown food. I could see that I would need to participate in this new way of life or else risk being shut out, isolated, and judged by the kids around me. So, I did.

Food became a thread that linked me both to Italy, where I'd spent my childhood, and to the States, where I now lived as a teenager. I could make espresso and froth the milk for a cappuccino by shaking it up in an empty bottle. I knew how to bake elegant tortes and roll out homemade puff pastry. I was a novelty. I cooked to hide my pain. I ate to hide my longing for home. I prepared traditional Italian dishes to impress others while filling my own body with Pop-Tarts, Twix, and Mountain Dew. I ate many American dishes for the first time: grilled cheese with ketchup, hamburgers, French fries, toaster waffles, and pancakes drenched in imitation maple syrup. I watched Saturday-morning cartoons while mindlessly devouring ready-bake cinnamon rolls from a can. Eating suddenly felt like an urgent, unpleasant act, with no time for timelessness. In Italy, food had been nourishment and medicine. In Kansas City, it became poison. I abandoned the practice of cooking and eating local, seasonal food for the sake of emotional survival at that time. However, it set up my digestive system for disaster when I spent time on the Indonesian island of Bali as a college student a few years later.

I only applied to one college: Middlebury College in Vermont. They accepted me and supported my vision to design my own major exploring how traditional people create reality with language and maintain that reality by sharing gastronomy through oral tradition. My studies brought me first to the Diné (Navajo) Reservation and then to Bali.

On Bali, I found, most people practiced some form of animism, a way of living that honors all beings and makes most daily activities into an offering. This includes the preparation, presentation, service, and solitary enjoyment of meals. Nourishment is sacred, and its relationship to each individual requires a ritual-like space. I learned this lesson while savoring an incredibly sweet rambutan fruit while riding the *bemo* (a small bus). That day, the six-passenger van-turned-bus was crammed with twelve people. They all stared at me in horror as I ate the delicious fruit.

When I asked one of my teachers why this had happened, she explained the role of food in Balinese culture. Food is seen as an offering to one another and the gods. Its consumption is private and personal, deserving space and respect. Those who do not eat in this way dishonor their bodies, the food, and the spirit realm. In that moment, I began to understand the importance of mindful eating. Later, when our student group visited a remote village in the Balinese rain forest, I mindfully accepted the food that was offered to me and ate it quietly while looking down at my plate. Though their water and electricity had been taken away by a cultural tourism construction project funded by the World Bank, the people in the village created an incredible feast over a simple fire—much as my uncle used to do in the Italian mountains.

I could never have imagined that this meal, eaten thoughtfully and with gratitude for our hosts, would change my life forever. That night, our group became extremely ill; vomiting, diarrhea, and fever overtook us all. We had come to expect that parasites were a part of life in the tropics, but no one had gotten quite this ill yet. We all took over-the-counter pills to expel parasites. After a few days, symptoms subsided.

I trusted that this was the end of that painful gut turmoil. But it was only the beginning. After finishing my studies in Indonesia, I traveled to Thailand and India before returning to the United States. When I arrived at my family's home in Kansas City, I turned on the faucet and poured myself a glass of water. I drank it, amazed at the fact that I could drink water straight from the tap. Then I filled my empty glass with milk and savored that as well—I had gone eight months without dairy products during my travels.

Little did I know that was the last time I would drink cow's milk. Within thirty minutes, I was on the floor, clutching my stomach and crying from the intensity of the cramping I felt. The experience reminded me of the period when I'd suffered from parasites while on Bali. The pain passed later that evening and I moved on, assuming it was an isolated incident. But I started noticing similar symptoms whenever I ate dairy, so I eventually I stopped eating it.

As time passed, more and more foods seemed to lead to gastrointestinal distress. Over the course of four years, I lost twenty pounds and my food choices became more restricted. My LDL cholesterol was elevated, my thyroid was sluggish, my stomach cramps persisted, I developed anxiety and depression, and my menstrual cycle stopped. As it turns out, these symptoms were my body's attempt to communicate with me, to indicate that systems were out of balance. But neither my Vermont family practitioner nor any of the specialists with whom I consulted had anything valuable to share besides affirming that I was "fine." They did not want to humor my reports of terrible ongoing symptoms and sent me away telling me to seek psychiatric counsel.

Health is a changing state that is different for everyone. This word has its root in many Indo-European languages, and that root means "holy" or "whole." I certainly did not feel whole. I felt fragmented and hollow.

A year later, I had the opportunity to be a patient for a Choctaw healer who was filming a healing ceremony for a shamanic studies museum in China. (I remain mesmerized by the fact that, to this day, there is a ceremony of me being healed playing over and over again for museum visitors in Shenzhen.) The day after the ceremony, the healer told me I had parasites, named the specific ones, and sent me to see a tropical disease specialist in Manhattan. That doctor confirmed her diagnosis: I had amebiasis, an infection caused by *Entamoeba histolytica*. These prehistoric parasites have strong cell walls that protect them from the stomach's acidic environment and allow them to burrow into the intestinal lining, ready to replicate. With a chronic infection like the one I was experiencing, the amoebas spread, colonizing outside my intestines, preying on my nervous system and liver.

The Manhattan doctor gave me two extremely potent antibiotics. After a few days of taking them, I felt like I was being poisoned, which I was. Antibiotics can eradicate a parasite after it is first contracted, but they can actually damage a system that suffers from chronic infection. Why? Because antibiotics destroy *all* intestinal bacteria, indiscriminately, including the beneficial ones that are fighting against colonies of parasites. They rid the intestines of their natural bacterial defenses and make more space for more parasites to flourish.

After that first noxious round of antibiotics, I attended a community dinner where I sat next to a friend of a friend who had just moved to town. He was an Ayurvedic practitioner, and we started talking about health. When I shared my story and amebiasis diagnosis, he directed me toward the parasite protocol in Paul Pitchford's *Healing with Whole Foods*. His recommendation felt more like a warning. He had had his own journey with parasites and explained that I would suffer tremendously if I did not do something other than take antibiotics. I took his words seriously, purchased the book, and began exploring traditional Chinese medicine. It became a pathway back to my own ancestral healing knowledge.

I was weak, shaky, and in constant pain. I could not sleep for more than three hours at a time and my anxiety was leading to panic attacks. I had developed disordered eating because I could not digest any food and felt uncomfortably full after eating just two or three bites of a meal. Food had always brought me such joy and played such a vital role in building a bridge of understanding with others. Now it was my greatest enemy, even though I needed it more than ever.

The war in my gut felt like it was escalating to a dramatic crescendo, and the parasites were winning. I felt poisoned. My vision was blurry, I could not drive, I was vomiting up most of my meals, and my intestines felt like they were on fire.

One hopeless morning, I recalled the simple, traditional foods I had been raised on. I thought about the recipes I learned growing up, passed down to me, my brother, and my cousins by my father, aunts, uncles, and grandmother. What made these foods so nourishing, so vitalizing, so life-giving? Each one contained seasonal ingredients with medicinal qualities, I realized. Deep down, I knew they could heal me.

This pivotal moment led me to explore the healing properties of olive oil, one of the cornerstone ingredients of my ancestral foodways. I discovered that oil from the first cold pressing of the olives is high in anti-inflammatory polyphenols, which reduce the risk of heart disease, maintain a balanced cholesterol profile, and reduce the overgrowth of ulcer-inducing *Helicobacter pylori* bacteria in the intestines. I was amazed to learn that olive oil—used in practically every dish with which I grew up—was an excellent tool for keeping intestinal parasites under control.

I realized that the antibiotics were simply clearing space in my intestines for the parasites to grow. I knew there had to be another way. I started taking two tablespoons daily of the first cold-press olive oil from an olive grove belonging to family friends in Tuscany. After two weeks, my gut cramping began to subside, like the oil was putting out a fire. My mindset switched from being the victim of a situation that was out of my control to being a student who was learning from my body's journey. I began to explore the use of essential oils in treating parasites. I added clove essential oil to my daily olive oil dose and found that my anxiety slowly receded.

There were many more steps on the journey to recovery, but remembering the use of ancestral food as medicine for my body, mind, and spirit was the beginning of my work to restore balance and move forward. As the years passed, I came to understand what controls hunger in the body, how to interpret cravings, and how to use the body's messages as tools for transformation. Simple, flavorful foods as close to the source as possible became my primary healers. I became grateful for my parents' annual visit to Vermont, when I could renew my connection with the foods and recipes with which they had raised me.

Whenever my parents visited, my father laced on his ancient hiking boots and headed to the south-facing hillsides in our local forests to forage for chanterelle mushrooms. After a bountiful harvest one summer, he and I cooked an immune-boosting lunch of risotto, an Italian staple that defines itself by its regional variations. In the south of Italy, risotto may be prepared with fresh tomatoes and seafood. A traditional northern recipe is made with minced onions, carrots, and celery sautéed in butter—a combination known as *soffritto*—with white wine and mixed with chanterelles. As we sat before the steaming bowls, we paused, and my father shared the prayer that his mother taught her children and grandchildren. Engaging with ancestral rituals and foods to reconnect to the place that defines our identity can feel grounding, calming, and nurturing, just a like a warm bowl of risotto.

🍎 Chanterelle Risotto

6 cups chicken stock

3 tablespoons butter

1 yellow onion, minced (about 1 cup)

½ teaspoon salt

2 stalks celery, minced

2 medium carrots, minced

½ pound fresh chanterelle mushrooms, diced*

2 cups risotto rice (Arborio or Carnaroli)†

½ cup white wine

¼ cup grated Parmigiano Reggiano (optional)

Bring the chicken stock to a gentle simmer in a pot.

Heat the butter in a deep skillet and add the onion. Cook over medium heat until it starts to brown, about 5 minutes. Add the salt as it cooks.

Add the celery and carrots and cook for a few more minutes.

Add the diced chanterelles and turn the heat to medium-high. Cook for 5 more minutes. Smell the earthy fragrance that rises from the cooking mushrooms. Offer a moment of praise for the endless network of mycelium that spans the forest, informing trees and ferns about woodland activity from miles away.

Stir in the rice and cook until it becomes translucent, about another 2 minutes. Add an extra handful of rice for an unexpected guest.

Pour in the white wine. Reduce the heat to medium-low.

At this point, stop stirring. I know that many people talk about stirring risotto constantly. I grew up never stirring it. I love the risotto my family prepares. Try it. It will work out.

Once the wine has been absorbed, start adding the hot stock, a ladle or two at a time. When you see bubbles rising to the surface of the rice, add another ladle or two of stock—just enough so that the stock barely covers the rice. Keep adding stock until the rice is cooked. My father swears it takes exactly 18 minutes.

Add the Parmigiano (if using), stir well, and serve a ladle or two to each person at the table. Eat steaming hot.

---

*Brush any dirt off the chanterelles before chopping them; do not wash them to maintain their flavor.

†Another way to measure the rice is to put a handful per person into the skillet.

Every traditional culture weaves food as medicine into daily life. Over time, with modernization, migration, and globalization, these daily food practices have changed or been forgotten. After my family moved to Kansas City, we found ourselves praying over hot dogs with supermarket pickled relish served on white buns. "God bless this food which now we take, and do us good for Jesus's sake. Amen." I remember glancing sidelong at my mom as my grandfather recited these words every evening at dinner. How could we be praying over this mass-market, industrially produced food that had no roots—no local provenance, no seasonality, no farmer or forager or maker to thank? I started trying to bring the same degree of quality and mindfulness I'd been accustomed to in Italy to the foods my American grandparents enjoyed. I started taking some of the foods that they ate to places like Loose Park, the local nature spot. It helped me restore my connection to myself as a member of the natural world and gave me solace in a world of denatured foods.

🍅 Late-Night Grilled Cheese

> 2 tablespoons (or more) pastured butter
> 2 slices good bread, preferably sourdough rye
> 3 slices Fontina cheese, or whatever variety is your favorite

Spread butter on each slice of bread.

Heat a skillet on the stove, preferably one that is cast iron or stainless steel. Turn the heat down to medium-low and place one slice of bread on it, butter side down. Hear it sizzle. Place the cheese on top of the sizzling bread.

Then place the second slice of bread on top of the cheese, butter side up.

Cook over low heat for a couple of minutes.

Flip the sandwich with a wide spatula. Press it down gently.

Listen to the butter melting. Breathe in the aroma of spring cow pastures, if you remember them.

Rip off a sheet of aluminum foil and lay it flat on the counter.

Check the bottom of the sandwich. When it is crisped to your liking, scoop out the sandwich and place it on the foil.

Wrap it up and take it to Loose Park after midnight. Tomorrow, Mom will chide you for leaving the dirty skillet on the stove.

Through my experience of using the foods of my heritage to heal myself of chronic infection, I began to understand how we are all indigenous to a place. Our gut microbiome reminds us of that whenever we try to digest food that our internal ecosystem is not familiar with. Of course, my heritage is not only Italian but also French, Welsh, and Polish. But I am most like my dad's sisters, and my body thrives when eating foods from the Mediterranean. I appreciate cabbage and potatoes from the northern European part of my ancestry, but they feel like occasional foods for me, as opposed to olives and fish, which feel like daily nourishment. And here in Vermont—an appreciably colder climate than the Mediterranean—I'm drawn to eat those northern European foods mainly in the winter.

When considering which foods best suit your daily nourishment, honor the mosaic of who you are. Notice which of your ancestors you most resemble, assess your current environment, and consider which parts of your ancestry resonate the most. It is not always easy to look at our heritage. I am not proud of some things my ancestors have done. For me, approaching ancestral healing through food has helped me accept the pain of my inheritance as a white, European colonist and to embrace the nourishing aspects of who I am. The following recipe, from the Mediterranean side of my heritage, expedited my healing.

🍅 Zuppa Verde: Italian Green Vegetable Soup

2 tablespoons olive oil

1 yellow onion, finely sliced

2 medium leeks, white and tender green parts, finely sliced

4 stalks celery, chopped

4 medium carrots, finely sliced

3 fingerling potatoes, diced

3 small, firm zucchini, sliced

3 cups chicken or vegetable stock

Salt, thyme, and sage, to taste

2 cups fresh green beans, tips snapped, broken into
    ½-inch lengths

Chopped fresh basil, for serving

Gently heat the olive oil in a soup pot. Add the onion and sauté for 10 minutes over low heat.

Add the leeks, celery, carrots, potatoes, and zucchini. Sauté for 5 more minutes. Add the stock, salt, thyme, and sage. Bring to a boil, then reduce the heat to medium and cook, covered, for about ½ hour.

Add the green beans and cook until they are tender but still a bit crunchy, about 15 minutes.

Add a handful of chopped fresh basil and serve.

The Songs Become My Home

I sing a song of two homes, raised
in a medieval city studded with cobblestones
where divination with tarocchi was born,
then taken to a cow town that croons middle America
where suburbs separate ranches and mansions
even though everyone goes to church bingo.
I sing a simple song so I will not forget
how pasta needs the freshest eggs
and bread is made from mother dough
with grain milled between stones
in a land of olive trees
that have reached to the sky for centuries.

FOOD AS A FOUNDATION FOR HEALTH

We each have unique life experiences, yet we are all connected by the shared understanding of what it's like to feel imbalance and restore balance. Change is the nature of reality. I share stories, research, books, articles, and ancestral wisdom in these pages. As the human experience changes, so will this information change. What may feel important now may no longer feel relevant in the future. However, every bit of information that I share is a building block in a process of the evolution of understanding. There are those who bow at the evidence-based altar of science; others prefer spiritual or religious practice. Despite their differences, both are ways to tread the path of the seeker. Whether we desire to deepen intellect, intuition, or both, scientific and spiritual pursuits arrive at the same conclusion: We are complex beings living in an increasingly complex world. Stepping away from binary, black-and-white thinking frees us up to be able to hold the complexity of life and the relativity of truth. Even the words in this book are lacking, forgetting, and trying their best to represent the elegant intricacy of the human experience during a moment in time. As you are exploring ways to transform, be open to the possibility that something you believe to be true right now can shift.

Why is traditional knowledge of nutrition and herbs as foundations of health missing from the modern biomedical curriculum? In 1910, the Carnegie Foundation hired Abraham Flexner, an educator and administrator who had studied at Johns Hopkins University, to write a report on medical education. This report led to government funding for biomedical research and pharmaceutical medications.[1] These advances put the United States on par with countries like Germany and the United Kingdom, which had previously dominated the biomedical research field. However, Flexner's report also caused many schools that had been focused on naturopathic, homeopathic, herbal, and chiropractic medicine to close. It led to a medical curriculum focused more on research and less on patient-centered whole health, including nutrition and coevolution with nature. Despite the 1960s movement toward integrating complementary and alternative medicine (CAM) into the biomedical curriculum, it was not until 1991 that the U.S. National Institutes of Health offered a small budget to create the National Center for Complementary and Alternative Medicine (NCCAM).

In 2014, I had the opportunity to work with the newly founded Goldring Center for Culinary Medicine at Tulane University School of Medicine in New Orleans. This was the first center of its kind to help medical residents learn about the foundational importance of nutrition in the health of their future patients. Since that time, the Goldring Center has brought its curriculum to more than thirty medical schools across the United States and Canada. Efforts such as these are bridging the gap created by the shift toward biomedical research after World War I and reintegrating food as medicine into doctors' toolkits. These efforts to bring a holistic, functional approach to medicine are key to preventing illness and minimizing dependence on pharmaceuticals. They empower us to use daily interventions such as food in our personal wellness plans so that we all depend less on an overburdened medical system and rely more on our bodies' messages for healing.

WHAT IS TRUE HUNGER?

How often do we feel genuinely hungry for food?

Hunger is the body's physiological response to unbalanced blood glucose. Blood glucose stabilizes when we take in nourishment. Our motivation to eat—becoming hungry, eating, feeling full, and then starting over—is controlled by the hunger hormone, ghrelin, and the satiety hormone, leptin. But this simple cycle is complicated by psychological associations with food.

We have strong associations, many of them from childhood, that connect food with specific activities, rituals, and even emotions. When we judge certain foods as unhealthy, they gain power and become more attractive. What if food did not involve judgment? This might mean that a slice of cake is sometimes a healthy choice, just as a bowl of broccoli is sometimes most supportive.

When I started my journey to heal myself of chronic intestinal parasites, I had developed both extreme cravings and intense aversions to certain foods. I craved the foods that feed parasites: sugar, flour, and dairy. I had aversions to foods that are harder to digest because my intestines were compromised by my unwanted guests. I had to rewire my brain and renourish my gut microbiome so that I could crave the foods I needed for healing. By eating more protein, fats, and vegetables, I changed my gut bacteria into the kind that can crowd out parasites instead of contributing to their proliferation. This shift took a great deal of awareness and patience. It began with understanding my motivations around food and eating.

To begin, I focused on consuming spices that traditionally help people maintain balanced intestinal flora and ward off illness. The following recipe felt supportive during my convalescence.

🍎 Soothing Vegetable Stew

    2 tablespoons olive oil
    2 cloves garlic, minced
    ¼ teaspoon ground cinnamon
    1 teaspoon ground cumin
    ½ teaspoon ginger
    ½ teaspoon ground turmeric
    2 onions, diced
    3 carrots, sliced
    2 pounds green cabbage, chopped
    2 sweet potatoes, chopped into 1-inch pieces
    ½ teaspoon salt
    4 cups chicken or vegetable broth

In a large skillet or frying pan, heat the oil over medium heat. Add the minced garlic along with the cinnamon, cardamom, cumin, ginger, and turmeric, then reduce the heat to low. Cook for just one minute, stirring once or twice.

Add the onions and sauté briefly, for 2 to 3 minutes.

Add the rest of the vegetables and sauté for 15 minutes. Add the salt and broth. Bring to a boil, then cover, reduce the heat, and simmer for 15 minutes. Enjoy.

The capacity to use food as medicine is rooted in observing the kinds of hunger we experience, tuning in to our intuition about why they occur, and learning how to support ourselves during those times. Sometimes we really do need to eat to fulfill a hunger; sometimes we need something else. The more I aligned with the medicinal qualities of the foods I was eating, the more I began to see my food cravings for what they were: information on how best to move forward.

The following types of association-driven hunger seem to be common to the human experience.

Scheduled Hunger

This happens when we are trying to eat on a schedule: The clock strikes noon and it's lunchtime, regardless of whether or not we are hungry. Many of us have been taught to eat at specific times of day, which confuses the body's hormonal hunger messages. Instead of watching the clock, it can be helpful to breathe into the moments when meals are typically scheduled and allow the body to communicate about whether it is hungry.

A sense of urgency to eat often comes after we have been hungry for some time. It's important to respond to hunger cues, like a growling stomach, before urgency sets in, regardless of the time of day. Depending on how we slept, what is happening in life, and the season, our daily eating rhythm may look different at different times.

Hunger by Association

This kind of hunger happens when we have created a particular pattern. I used to eat dark chocolate after dinner. Some of us like to eat popcorn while watching television or snack on trail mix while hiking. These associations are wonderfully satisfying . . . until we start to find that they no longer serve us. When I realized that my challenges in falling asleep were related to the chocolate, I was motivated to stop eating it in association with the end of a meal. Instead, I started brewing myself a pot of tea made with relaxing herbs after dinner.

Pay attention to times when these different kinds of hunger come up in your day. Awareness precedes change.

Emotional Hunger

Emotional hunger is triggered by feelings such as overwhelm and exhaustion. Emotional eating is a way to process feelings through eating. If this act feels helpful in the moment, please engage in it. Sometimes, eating our feelings is exactly what's needed. If you prefer an alternative, notice the emotions that are present when you are called to eat emotionally. Find another outlet for digesting your emotions, such as movement, deep breathing, or a conversation with a loved one.

ABOUT CRAVINGS

When we reach for a treat or crave a certain food, what do we really need? Try to stop, take a breath, and ask yourself this question before you eat. Sometimes you might just need water, movement, fresh air, or rest. Cravings can be authentic messages from the body asking for nourishment, or they can be related to emotional, scheduled, or associative hunger. The more we listen to the body, the more we can discern which kind of craving is happening.

Serotonin is one of the body's primary happiness hormones. If serotonin levels are low, we tend to feel sad. The gut plays a key role in managing the body's hormones. When we feel off balance, gut flora send messages to the brain, telling it to generate a sugar or carbohydrate craving. Eating sugar or carbohydrates gives us a brief burst of serotonin. However, that food-based happiness is fleeting because it does not actually help the body produce the amount of serotonin needed to balance mood. This form of emotional hunger simply exacerbates nervous system dysregulation instead of helping to manage it.

Fat and protein can be helpful nutrients to bring the nervous system back into balance. These nutrients do not require as much insulin as carbohydrates to be digested, so blood glucose remains more stable when consuming them. When the body produces too much insulin in response to high levels of glucose from carbohydrates and sugars in the bloodstream, the brain reduces the amount of serotonin it produces. Serotonin is one of the body's feel-good hormones. If serotonin declines, gut bacteria signal the brain to crave more carbohydrates and sugars, and the cycle repeats itself. However, if glucose-producing foods are eaten alongside protein and/or fat, the brain doesn't down-regulate serotonin production.

So, when my kids ask me for bread and butter, I offer it to them on a plate alongside an Energy Bite made with nuts and seeds that are high in fat and protein (you can find the recipe on page 180). Their bodies will metabolize the bread more slowly thanks to the presence of nuts and seeds.

Excessively sweet foods, like those with refined sugar from sugar beets and sugar cane, trigger the release of endorphins, which stimulate the pleasure center of the brain. This is why many nutritionists consider refined sugar to be an addictive chemical rather than a food.

Here are some ways to cultivate joy and embrace cravings that don't involve highly processed industrial food:

Savor the sweet flavor. Enjoy sweet foods that are unprocessed, such as roasted carrots or sweet potatoes. In the evening, if you're craving a sweet dessert but feel like the sugar will keep you up, enjoy cooked blueberries or apples with cinnamon and cardamom, or have a warm cup of coconut milk or almond milk with a pinch of nutmeg.

Drink water. Try to notice how much water you need to drink daily to feel satisfied. If you notice thirst, it's time to drink more water. Add lemon juice to change the flavor experience or salt to restore electrolytes if you have been sweating or if you are very thirsty.

Move your body. When a craving hits or an emotional wave overtakes you, walk away! Try to make funny faces, swing your arms around, go for a brief walk, put on some music, or lay down on the floor and move your limbs in any way that feels intuitively supportive.

Get good sleep. Getting seven to eight hours of sleep per night improves immunity and gives us greater capacity to recognize and interpret cravings. Try to stop eating two hours before bed so that all your food has passed through your stomach before you sleep. Try to go to bed by 10:00 p.m. If you experience nocturnal hypoglycemia (low blood glucose while sleeping), have a snack high in protein and fat, such as Energy Bites (see page 180 for the recipe), to support you as you sleep.

Transforming Cravings

Do you tend to crave a certain type of food? Is this craving supportive or counterproductive? In his book *Tiny Habits,* Stanford behavioral psychologist B. J. Fogg talks about how we can shift our behavior through "baby steps"—that is, cultivating small changes in our habits. If we apply that concept to the idea of using food as medicine, we can start by noticing which foods feel nourishing and supportive and which foods don't. We can start to build beneficial eating habits by also bringing our awareness to the ways we eat: When we eat, which environments and practices are grounding and fulfilling, and which are not?

When I was healing myself of intestinal parasites, I had to reintroduce many foods that I had avoided for years. I needed to expand my eating so I could gain weight and strength and diversify my nutrient intake. However, I hung on to my restrictive way of eating for a long time because, even though it was not serving me any longer, its familiarity was comforting. As I slowly let go, I gave myself the courage to try new foods by thanking each one that came across my plate.

This gratitude practice started small and grew as my confidence increased. As I started enjoying more foods without crippling gut pain, I felt stronger, more vibrant, and less anxious. When I made this shift toward a mindset of gratitude, I began to reach for the things that brought me joy. It may sound simple, but switching our mindset in this way is essential to shifting our habits. When we do not love and appreciate ourselves, we are more likely to continue perpetuating old habits because we are unconsciously avoiding growth.

On the flip side, sometimes we need to eliminate certain foods from our eating—and that can be challenging. Sometimes we give in to cravings and eat foods we know we should avoid. That simply means that we are human. The gut microbiome is adapted to digest the foods we have been eating. When they are deprived of those foods, gut bacteria send messages to the brain, triggering cravings. To change the strains of bacteria in our gut and stop those cravings, we first change what we eat, and we must wait as the old strains are eliminated and new strains begin to take over. This is a process of self-transformation. As with any journey, it is not linear, and it calls for compassion.

Cravings as Information

Do you ever have cravings that seem to come out of nowhere? According to traditional Chinese medicine and Ayurveda, these sudden cravings are the body's way of communicating specific needs. In Chinese medicine, these messages relate to the organ systems and seasons (see chapter 3); in Ayurveda, they relate to the pitta, kapha, and vata doshas, or constitutions (see chapter 2).

Cravings for sweets, grains, and other carbohydrates might mean that the body and mind are working hard or that the heart is not feeling nourished; digestion may be weak and we may be struggling to manage stress. These cravings correlate to the stomach and spleen time of late summer in Chinese medicine, which is pitta (fire) time in the Ayurvedic tradition.

Cravings for pungent, spicy foods indicate that the immune system is weakened or overworked. It also indicates that sorrow and grief need to be expressed. These correlate to the lung and large intestine time of autumn in Chinese medicine, which is the transition to vata (wind) time in the Ayurvedic tradition.

Cravings for salt and salty flavors like chips or hard cheese signal fear, kidney issues, and water imbalance (bloating or dehydration). These match up with the kidney and bladder time of winter in Chinese medicine, which is vata (wind) time in the Ayurvedic tradition.

Cravings for sour flavors like citrus, vinegar, and lemonade signal anger, stress, frustration, and indigestion. These match up with the liver and gallbladder time of spring in Chinese medicine, which is kapha (earth) time in the Ayurvedic tradition.

Cravings for bitter flavors like coffee, dark chocolate, tobacco, alcohol, and dark leafy greens signal mental restlessness, a need for stimulation, and a need for cardiovascular support. These correlate with the heart and small intestine time of summer in Chinese medicine, which is pitta (fire) time in the Ayurvedic tradition.

Notice any of these cravings and give them special attention during their season.

When I found myself craving carbohydrates, I started baking one of my favorite childhood comfort foods in a more digestible form. A staple of Italian-Austrian cuisine, the sourdough soft pretzel is so iconic in Bressanone that my family's favorite local bakery, Mutschlechner (try to say that three times fast), has a wrought-iron pretzel hanging outside as a shop sign.

🍅 Sourdough Pretzels

> 1 cup Quinoa Sourdough Starter (page 116)
> 1 cup arrowroot flour
> 2 cups almond flour, plus a bit for rolling the dough
> ¼ cup ground flaxseed meal
> ¼ teaspoon salt
> 1 cup coconut milk (or whatever milk you prefer)
> 3 tablespoons coconut oil or ghee, melted
> 2 tablespoons baking soda, for boiling the pretzels
> Coarse or flaky salt, for sprinkling on top
> 1 egg, beaten, for brushing the pretzels

Before bed, mix the starter, arrowroot flour, almond flour, flaxseed meal, salt, milk, and oil/ghee together in a mixing bowl. Cover with a cloth and leave on the counter overnight. The next morning, make the pretzels.

Cover your hands in almond flour and sprinkle some on a cutting board. Then divide the dough into seven balls.

Roll out a ball into a rope on the cutting board. Bring each end of the rope toward you to make a horseshoe shape. Twist the ends of the rope together twice. Then bring them over the top of the horseshoe. Press the two ends down onto the curve. (You may need to wet the ends a bit with water to get them to stick.)

Repeat with the other six balls.

Meanwhile, bring a large pot of water to a boil. Add the baking soda.

Preheat the oven to 425°F and line a baking sheet with parchment paper.

Crack an egg into a bowl and beat it lightly. Get some coarse or flaky salt ready.

Once the water is boiling, add two or three pretzels. As soon as one floats to the top (which should take about 30 seconds), scoop it out with a slotted spoon and place it on the baking sheet.

Repeat until all the pretzels have been boiled.

Then, brush them all with egg, sprinkle them with salt, and bake them for 18 minutes, or until they are golden brown.

Enjoy the pretzels dipped in stone-ground mustard alongside soft-boiled eggs for breakfast while ruminating on the power of mountains to reveal the ancient topography of the sea floor.

Food as medicine is rooted both in what we eat and in how we eat it. Enjoying our food is essential to digesting and assimilating it effectively. The more we enjoy life, the more we enjoy food. When I returned to the foods with which I grew up as tools for healing, I began to thrive. The anxiety, depression, insomnia, and gut pain that I experienced for years started to fade into the background. I realized that, for me, the foundations of health are nonjudgment, compassion, and surrender to change.

2

Constitution Informs Nourishment

Ayurveda, Chinese Five Element Theory, and the Mediterranean Way

One who indulges daily in healthy foods and activities,
who discriminates the good and bad of everything and then
acts wisely, who is not attached too much to the objects of
the senses, who develops the habit of charity, of considering
all as equal, of truthfulness, of pardoning and keeping
company of good persons, becomes free from all diseases.

ASHTANGA HRIDAYAM

I was sitting in a classroom of forty students in Albuquerque, New Mexico. We were all eager to learn from Dr. Vasant Lad, the lineage carrier of the Ayurvedic tradition. As he taught us about this ancient, unbroken healing tradition from his native India, Dr. Lad asked us if we could identify our own prakriti, or the constitution with which we were born. Based on extensive study, I identified myself as both pitta, a fire type, and kapha, an earth type. We went around the circle and each student stated their constitution. When it was my turn, Dr. Lad looked at me inquisitively. Then he called me up to the front of the room. He asked if I could show him my tongue and let him listen to my pulse.

After doing so, he looked at me with a twinkle in his eye. "Parasites," he said, nodding gently. Then he turned to the class and explained that, even though I presented as more of vata, an air type, I did indeed have fire and earth in my constitution. Because I had suffered from a chronic parasitic infection for ten years, my constitution had been dramatically altered. This complexity of the combination between the constitution with which we are born and the conditions that affect us over the course of our lives is at the intersection of food and health.

The more we can appreciate just how unique we all are and how different our life circumstances can be, the more we understand how the healing process is specific to each one of us. Healing traditions worldwide have common roots. There is a great deal of inherited complexity that many of us must unpack. The more we look at our ancestry and uncover which systems of wellness align with our heritage, the more we understand the intersectionality of the human experience and the importance of understanding our personal histories in the journey toward equity. We are part of nature, and these ways of healing reveal this intrinsic truth: Earth is our ultimate ancestor, equalizer, and guide toward collective liberation.

My life and studies have guided me to deepen my knowledge of three traditional healing philosophies: Ayurveda (from the Sanskrit *ayus*, life, and *veda*, knowledge), Chinese five element theory, and the Mediterranean way, which is based in Greco-Roman traditional healing.* These philosophies offer a framework for observing and learning from patterns as they unfold in every part of nature.

---

*Throughout this book I have avoided use of the word *diet* as a generalized way of eating—such as the "Mediterannean diet"—wherever possible because of the negative connotations now associated with this word. Instead you will see that I use "Mediterannean way" or "way of eating" and other similar phrasing to represent the same meaning. More on the true meaning of *diet* and its current usage and connotations in our culture in the Intuitive Eating section (see page 89).

AYURVEDA

Ayurveda (आयुर्वेद in Sanskrit) is a centuries-old healing modality from the Indian subcontinent that encompasses all realms of health, from emotional and physical to spiritual and psychological. In Ayurvedic theory, like increases like: When the weather is more dry (as it often is in winter), our bodies are also more dry.

Food is seen as therapeutic nourishment, and Ayurveda offers health-related dietary guidelines, though traditional dishes can vary widely between regions—which is no surprise, given the diverse ethnicities and geography of the region. One teaching is constant, though, and Dr. Lad explained it well: "Eat when you're hungry, drink when you're thirsty, sleep when you're tired." In other words, heed your natural urges. Following this adage, in conjunction with understanding our inherent constitution, can provide guidance for maintaining wellness through life's changes.

Ayurvedic Constitution
Prakriti (प्रकृति I in Sanskrit) is our unique constitution. The word prakriti means original, fundamental, from the source. Our prakriti is determined when we are conceived and is comprised of genetically inherited physical and emotional qualities. It relates to those characteristics that are fairly constant in our being. While we may experience temporary changes, like gaining or losing weight or having a cold, we will never experience a dramatic change in eye color or skin tone. Constitution is seen through the lens of doshas (दोषः in Sanskrit), or mind-body types. Each of us has all three doshas in our constitution, in unique proportions.

The three doshas are:

Vata (वात): air or wind
Pitta (पतित्): fire or bile
Kapha (कफ): earth or phlegm

What Is Your Constitution?

Knowing your prakriti, or constitution, can help you maintain optimal health. Answer the questions below based on your overall, lifelong tendencies, not according to temporary or recent conditions. Use the following scale: 1—does not apply; 2—somewhat applies; 3—applies.

1. During my life, I have tended toward being thin.
2. I find maintaining daily routines to be challenging.
3. My skin tends to be rough and dry, even if I don't live in a dry climate.
4. My joints are prominent.
5. My teeth are protruding and/or crooked.
6. My hair is curly and tends to be dry or frizzy.
7. It is easy for me to lose weight and I have difficulty gaining weight.
8. I tend to enjoy hot weather.
9. I tend to dislike wind.
10. I tend to dislike dry weather.
11. I have a medium build with medium bones.
12. I enjoy competitive activities and intellectual challenges.
13. My teeth are medium-sized and/or yellow.
14. I have fair skin and I sunburn easily.
15. I have a lot of moles or freckles.
16. I am or am becoming bald, I have grayed early, or I have fine hair.
17. Chile peppers, tomatoes, and spicy food give me heartburn, stomachache, or loose stools.
18. I prefer a cool climate to a warm one.
19. I dislike heat, especially humid heat, and feel easily fatigued by it.
20. I have a sharp, intelligent mind.
21. I have a sturdy constitution and large bones.
22. I tend toward being at least a little overweight.
23. My teeth are large, straight, and white.

24. My hair is a thick and lustrous.

25. My eyes are large and luxurious.

26. I can easily sleep for 8 to 10 hours per night.

27. I gain weight easily and have a hard time losing it.

28. I tend to have excess mucus.

29. I tolerate most climates, but I prefer hot, dry weather.

30. My energy and stamina are consistent.

Working by sections, add up the numbers to determine your predominant traits.

- Questions 1–10 are vata-focused; high scores here reflect a light, subtle nature.
- Questions 11–20 are pitta-focused; high scores here reflect a bright, fiery nature.
- Questions 21–30 are kapha-focused; high scores here reflect a grounded, steady nature.

Note: This test cannot take the place of an evaluation by a qualified Ayurvedic practitioner. This evaluation is based on teachings from Dr. Vasant Lad at the Ayurvedic Institute.

Foods to Balance the Doshas

The ideal state is one of balance among the three doshas. If a particular dosha predominates in your constitution, you can use foods/tastes that decrease that dosha to restore balance. Use the lists below as a starting point, keeping in mind that they do not name *all* the foods that decrease each dosha.

Note: You will not find any meats on these lists of food. Ayurveda considers meat to be a therapeutic food during times of convalescence. It is seen as an appropriate food for cold weather, for recovery from illness, and for those who intuitively feel strengthened by it.

Vata Foods

Vata is cool, dry, and light. The pungent, bitter, and astringent tastes increase vata by increasing its drying and cooling qualities. The sweet, sour, and salty tastes decrease vata by bringing moisture, bulk, and warmth to the body, which are opposite qualities to those of vata.

Eat foods that are warm, moist, oily, and nourishing to balance the vata in your constitution. Some examples include:

Fruit: apples (cooked), bananas, berries, coconuts, dates, figs, grapes, kiwis, lemons, papayas, peaches, plums

Vegetables: asparagus, avocados, beets, carrots, garlic, green beans, leeks, mustard greens, parsnips, pumpkins, spinach, sweet potatoes, winter squash

Nuts and seeds (soak before eating to improve digestibility): almonds, cashews, pecans, pine nuts, walnuts, pumpkin seeds, sesame seeds, sunflower seeds

Grains: amaranth, oats, rice

Legumes: lentils, mung beans

Dairy (if tolerated): butter, raw cheese, cottage cheese, yogurt

Sweeteners: date sugar, honey, molasses

Oils: avocado oil, coconut oil, ghee, olive oil, sesame oil, sunflower oil

Pitta Foods

Pitta is oily, sharp, hot, and light. Pungent, sour, and salty tastes increase pitta by increasing its hot quality. Sweet, bitter, and astringent tastes decrease pitta by providing the opposite qualities to those of pitta.

Eat foods that are mild, cooling, and grounding to balance the pitta in your constitution. Some examples include:

Fruits: apples, apricots, berries, coconuts, dates, figs, grapes, limes, mangos, melons, oranges, papayas, plums, pomegranates, raisins, watermelons

Vegetables: asparagus, avocados, beets, bell peppers, broccoli, Brussels sprouts, cabbages, carrots, cauliflower, celery, cilantro, collard greens, cucumbers, green beans, leeks, lettuce, mushrooms, okra, olives, onions, potatoes, spinach, sprouts, summer and winter squashes, sweet potatoes, tapioca, zucchini

Nuts and seeds: almonds, flax seeds, pumpkin seeds, sunflower seeds

Grains: amaranth, barley, oats, quinoa, rice

Legumes: adzuki beans, black-eyed peas, garbanzo beans, kidney beans, lentils, mung beans

Dairy (if tolerated): butter, cottage cheese, goat cheese

Sweeteners: date syrup, maple syrup

Oils: coconut oil, flax oil, ghee, olive oil, walnut oil

Kapha Foods

Kapha is heavy, cool, and oily. The sweet, sour, and salty tastes increase kapha by increasing bulk and moisture in the body and mind, perpetuating the qualities of kapha. The pungent, bitter, and astringent tastes decrease kapha by drying the body and providing the opposite qualities to those of kapha.

Choose foods that are light, warm, and dry to balance the kapha in your constitution. Some examples include:

Fruit: apples, apricots, berries, grapes, lemons, mangos, peaches, pears, persimmons, pomegranates, raisins

Vegetables: artichokes, asparagus, beets, bell peppers, broccoli, burdock roots, cabbages, carrots, cauliflower, celery, chiles, daikon radishes, eggplants, garlic, green beans, kale, leafy greens, leeks, mustard greens, onions, peas, potatoes, radishes, spinach, tapioca, tomatoes, winter squashes

Nuts and seeds: almonds, chia seeds, flax seeds, pumpkin seeds

Grains: amaranth, buckwheat, couscous, millet, oats, polenta, quinoa, rice

Legumes: adzuki beans, lentils, mung beans

Dairy (if tolerated): cottage cheese, goat cheese, yogurt
Sweeteners: honey
Oils: flax oil, ghee, sunflower oil

What Is Ghee?

Ghee is clarified butter: unsalted butter that has been separated from its water and milk proteins. It is considered a dairy-free food in Ayurveda and is lubricating, soothing, and supportive. When heated, butter separates into three layers: the casein, a frothy layer on top; the clarified fat (ghee) in the middle; and the milk solids and proteins at the bottom.

♠ Ghee

Heat I pound of unsalted butter in a stainless-steel stock pot. When it starts bubbling, reduce the heat to low.

Fetch a small bowl and spoon.

Stay with the butter, skimming the foamy white casein that rises to the surface with the spoon. Keep skimming for about 15 minutes, or until the ghee has stopped talking with its bubbling sounds.

As you watch your butter separate, notice the constellations that swirl in the rising the milk solids. You may want to save the casein and mix it into a pot of cooking rice.

Send a prayer to the cows that grazed on green summer grass and golden winter hay to offer the milk that made this butter. Cows are considered sacred in Ayurvedic tradition for a reason: the nourishing fat that comes from these powerful and peaceful animals is a healing balm for all doshas.

As soon as the ghee is no longer speaking to you, remove it from the heat. Strain through a fine-mesh tea strainer or cheesecloth into a glass jar. This process removes leftover milk solids.

Allow it to cool completely before closing the jar.

Ghee will keep at room temperature for 2 to 3 weeks.

Eating to Balance Each Dosha

Ayurveda sees each element as corresponding with constitutional traits, times of life, and times of each year. Childhood is considered kapha time, the earth element. Mid-life is pitta time, the fire element. Elders are seen as being in vata time, the air element. With the seasons, winter correlates with vata time as it tends to be windy. Spring is kapha time, representing the heaviness that can occur in the body when the earth is awakening. Summer is pitta time, the hottest time of year. When we have a predominant dosha that is activated because of the season, it can feel supportive to eat foods that pacify that dosha.

For most of us, more than one dosha predominates our individual constitutions. I am a pitta (fire) and kapha (earth) type. Thus, it is helpful for me to pay extra attention to the seasons in which my constitutional doshas are increased by the dosha of a certain time of year. In the spring, which is kapha time, I try to minimize oils and sweeteners, which are heavy, cool, and oily, since these promote kapha and are thus harder for kapha types to digest. In the summer, which is pitta time, I try to avoid foods that are oily, sharp, and spicy because they increase pitta. Instead, I enjoy cooling foods like cucumber, mint, and amaranth.

An important dish in the Ayurvedic tradition is kitchari, whose name means mixture, usually in reference to a mixture of a grain and a legume. Kitchari is considered deeply nourishing and easy for all constitutions to digest. Ayurvedic practitioners recommend spending three to five days each spring and fall eating kitchari for all meals. It is a gentle, simple nutritional reset that can help realign the organ systems.

Below you'll find my recipe for kitchari, followed by recipes that can help balance an excess of air (vata: gas and bloating), fire (pitta: heartburn and loose stools), or earth (kapha: fatigue and constipation).

♠ Kitchari

For the rice:

    1 cup long-grain brown rice

    2 cups water

    1 tablespoon ghee or coconut oil

    ¼ teaspoon salt

    1 teaspoon whole cumin seed

    1 teaspoon mustard seed

    ½ teaspoon ground coriander

    ½ teaspoon ground cumin

    1 teaspoon ground turmeric

    Chopped vegetables, such as asparagus, broccoli, cauliflower, collards, kale, spinach, summer squash, or zucchini (choose 2)

For the dahl:

    2 cups split yellow lentils

    6 cups water

    2–3 tablespoons ghee or coconut oil

    ½ teaspoon salt

    ½ teaspoon ground cumin

    1 teaspoon garam masala

    ½ teaspoon ground coriander

    ½ teaspoon ground turmeric

    Chopped vegetables, such as beets, carrots, parsnips, rutabaga, winter squash, or sweet potatoes (choose 2)

Begin with the rice: Rinse the rice. Transfer the rice to a pot and add the water. Bring to a boil, then reduce the heat and simmer, with the lid ajar, for 30 minutes.

In a skillet, heat the ghee or coconut oil with the salt, cumin and mustard seeds, and ground spices. When the seeds start popping, turn off the heat and pour the mixture into the cooking rice.

Add vegetables—asparagus, broccoli, cauliflowers, peas, squash, zucchini—to the rice while it is cooking.

To make the dahl, rinse the lentils. Transfer the dahl to a pot and add 5 cups of the water. Bring to a boil, then reduce the heat to medium and cook, uncovered, for 30 minutes, stirring occasionally. Skim off any white foam that develops and discard it.

In a skillet, heat the ghee or coconut oil with the salt, cumin, garam masala, coriander, and turmeric.

Add vegetables, such as beets, carrots, collards, kale, spinach, and sweet potatoes, to the skillet. Add the remaining 1 cup water and cooked lentils. Cover, and simmer over low heat for 15 minutes. Mix into the rice, stir, and enjoy.

♠ Vata-Balancing Greens

3 cups vegetable or chicken broth

3 cups mustard greens, chopped

2 packed cups spinach, chopped

2 teaspoons chile flakes

½ teaspoon salt

3 tablespoons ghee

¾-inch piece of fresh ginger, minced

¼ teaspoon ground cinnamon

¼ teaspoon ground coriander

¼ teaspoon ground cumin

Heat the broth in a pot to a boil. Add the mustard greens and spinach, reduce the heat, and simmer for about 10 minutes.

Stir in the chile flakes and salt. Set aside.

In a skillet, warm the ghee and add the ginger, cinnamon, coriander, and cumin. Cook over low heat until the spices become fragrant, about 1 minute.

Add the spices to the cooked greens and stir well to incorporate. Simmer for 10 minutes more. Serve hot with cooked rice.

♠ Pitta-Balancing Dahl

    1 cup basmati rice

    ½ cup mung beans

    ⅓ cup chopped fresh cilantro

    2 tablespoons unsweetened shredded coconut

    ¾-inch piece of fresh ginger, minced

    2 tablespoons ghee

    ½ teaspoon salt

    ½ teaspoon ground turmeric

    ½ teaspoon ground coriander

    ¼ teaspoon ground cardamom

    4½ cups water

Rinse the rice and mung beans separately. Soak the mung beans in water for 2 hours, then drain.

Put the coconut, cilantro, ginger, and ½ cup of the water into a food processor and blend until liquefied.

Heat the ghee over medium heat in a large saucepan, Add the blended coconut mixture, along with the coriander, cardamom, salt, and turmeric. Stir well and bring to a boil to release the flavor.

Mix in the rice, mung beans, and remaining 4 cups of water. Return to a boil. Boil, uncovered, for 5 minutes. Then cover, leaving the lid slightly ajar, reduce the heat, and simmer for 30 minutes, until the beans and rice are tender.

♠ Kapha-Balancing Stew

    4 cups chopped cauliflower

    1 head broccoli, chopped

    5 cups vegetable broth

    2 tablespoons ghee

    ½ teaspoon salt

    ½ teaspoon ground cinnamon

1 teaspoon ground coriander

½ teaspoon ground fenugreek

1 teaspoon ground turmeric

½ teaspoon freshly ground black pepper

Combine the cauliflower and broccoli with the broth in a pot. Cook over low heat for about 20 minutes. Set aside.

In a skillet, warm the ghee. Add the salt and spices and cook over low heat until they become fragrant, 1 to 2 minutes.

Add the ghee and spices to the vegetables. Mash with a potato masher until the texture becomes thick.

Building Agni

The Sanskrit word *agni* means fire. In Ayurveda, it refers to digestive fire. It's important to have just the perfect amount of agni so that we can digest our food well without getting overheated. I learned agni-building recipes for pickles and chutneys from Dr. Lad while studying at the Ayurvedic Institute. These delicious foods stimulate digestion and balance overall metabolism. You can enjoy them alongside your meals as condiments. The pickles are appropriate for all constitutions and especially helpful when a meal feels heavy or digestion feels sluggish. The chutney can feel soothing to pitta types in particular and may work for vata types only in the summer.

♠ Ginger Lime Pickles

A thick piece of fresh ginger

Coarse sea salt

1 lime

Slice the ginger as thinly as possible with a sharp knife. Place the slices on a plate in one flat layer. Sprinkle them with coarse salt. Cut open the lime and squeeze it over the ginger. Let the slices sit for 5 minutes or so before eating.

You can make a jar of these and store them in the fridge, where they will keep for 3 days. Enjoy one before each meal.

♠ Coconut Cilantro Chutney

½ cup water
½ cup unsweetened shredded coconut
½ teaspoon sea salt
Juice of I lime
Freshly chopped cilantro (½ bunch)
Freshly chopped mint (½ bunch)

Combine all the ingredients in a food processor. Blend at the highest speed for 2 minutes.

Enjoy a spoonful along with your meal. Store the chutney in the refrigerator, where it will keep for a week.

CHINESE FIVE ELEMENT THEORY

If we can recognize health as a changing state of balance, then we can see illness, pain, and food cravings as signals of the body's disharmony. Chinese five element theory or traditional Chinese medicine (TCM), an ancient healing modality that persists today with doctors, naturopaths, and acupuncturists, regards food as medicine and provides the foundation to support balance. TCM sees the world as interconnected: five seasons are connected with five flavors, five emotions, and concomitant organ systems. The five elements begin with spring's rebirth and the wood element. Summer follows with the fire element. Late summer is earth time. Autumn embodies the metal element and winter is water.

The Five Flavors

The five elements correspond to five flavors: wood is sour, fire is bitter, earth is sweet, metal is pungent, and water is salty. To satisfy the whole being and maintain balance, TCM encourages the inclusion of all five flavors in each meal. Illness occurs when a flavor is used in excess.

The five flavors also correspond to the seasons: sweet for late summer, sour for fall, salty for winter, pungent for spring, and bitter for summer. When we cook with foods that match the season, we are healing ourselves and aligning with the Earth's process of cyclical change. Most foods have more than one flavor. Horseradish is sour and also pungent. Chicken is sour and also salty. These food examples are listed by their predominant action in the body.

Foods of the Five Flavors

Sweet (tonic, strengthening): carrots, sweet potatoes, winter squash, dates, honey, barley, oats, rice

Sour (astringent): horseradish, lemons, tomatoes, chicken, sauerkraut, vinegar, sourdough bread

Salty (purgative, grounding): eggs, beans, seaweed, miso, tamari, umeboshi plum

Pungent (promotes perspiration and circulation): ginger, onion, pepper, scallions, buckwheat

Bitter (cooling, moist): celery, unsweetened cocoa, dandelion, kale, olives, amaranth, millet, quinoa

When I started learning about TCM, I returned to cooking with the seasons. I remembered how seasonal foods influenced my family's meals when I was growing up, and I became inspired to experiment with different ingredients. I learned to substitute foods that tend to cause inflammation, like eggplants, peppers, tomatoes, corn, soy, wheat, and dairy, with foods that tend to be more soothing, like artichokes, coconuts, pumpkins, lentils, millet, and oats.

During my years of chronic illness, the principles of TCM supported me, not only in learning new ways to make food flavorful and nourishing, but also in understanding my own constitution and its imbalances as a tool for healing myself. Every time I changed a recipe to include all the five flavors, both my gut and my nervous system benefitted. I noticed that I was able to digest more food at a given meal and I felt calmer and more satisfied after eating. As I incorporated suggestions about sleep, movement, and other daily practices to nourish my constitution, I felt my vital essence returning to me, like a fire being rekindled after a long night.

The Nine Constitutions

In Chinese medicine, as Zhang Yifang and Yao Yingzhi explain in *Your Guide to Health with Foods and Herbs,* body constitution consists of "the characteristics of an individual, including structural and functional characteristics, temperament, adaptability to environmental changes and susceptibility to disease. It is relatively stable, being in part, genetically determined and in part, acquired."[1] TCM body constitutions are like the doshas of Ayurveda. As with the doshas, understanding your TCM constitution will help you choose foods with the goal of providing the body with the support it needs to restore balance.

If you identify with a constitution whose description includes the word *deficiency,* do not see it as a form of judgment. That word comes from the Latin *de* and *facere,* meaning "to do in reverse." Someone who is yang deficient simply needs to reverse that condition by cultivating expansive yang energy, which was perhaps depleted by life circumstances. Realizing that something like depletion has occurred is a blessing because it offers an opportunity for restoring harmony.

According to Yifang and Yingzhi, the nine body constitutions are:

Neutral 平和
Qi deficiency 氣虛
Yang deficiency 陽虛
Yin deficiency 陰虛
Blood stasis 血瘀
Phlegm-dampness 痰濕
Dampness-heat 濕熱
Qi stagnation 氣鬱
Intrinsic 特稟[2]

In Chinese medicine, as in Ayurveda, constitution affects how we feel and behave as well as how we respond to illness. These nine constitutions can change and interplay with one another. Each of us might have a combination of several of them, and as we change over

time, our body constitution also shifts. The more we work to harmonize our constitution, the closer we come to achieving the neutral
constitution.

Neutral Constitution

People with this constitution tend to have a radiant complexion and feel
adaptable thanks to an internal reservoir of energy.

To restore and maintain balance:

- Stay positive.
- Eat more frequent, smaller meals.
- Avoid foods that are oily or spicy.
- Take a brief walk after meals.

Qi Deficiency

People with this constitution feel tired or breathless and sweat when
feeling nervous or anxious.

To restore and maintain balance:

- Eat grounding foods, like animal protein.
- Avoid excessive amounts of raw food.
- Try to always stay warm.
- Take shelter from the wind.

Yang Deficiency

People with this constitution tend to have cold hands and feet, indigestion, and frequent colds.

To restore and maintain balance:

- Eat warming foods, like beef and onions.
- Avoid cold, raw foods.
- Keep the feet, back, and belly warm.
- Be gentle when exercising.
- Find activities that inspire joy.

Yin Deficiency

People with this constitution tend to feel irritable, have sore throats, and struggle with hot, dry weather.

To restore and maintain balance:

- Eat soothing, cooling foods, like coconut.
- Avoid drying foods, like nuts and corn.
- Try to go to bed before 10 p.m.
- Take a short walk to clear the mind.

Blood Stasis

People with this constitution tend to have dark circles under the eyes, dry skin, and frequent bruising.

To restore and maintain balance:

- Eat foods that support the liver, such as beans, seaweed, parsley, and bitter greens.
- Avoid animal products.
- Find activities that feel calming, such as deep breathing.
- Move the body in small, frequent bursts.

Phlegm-Dampness

People with this constitution likely experience an aversion to damp climates and inertia or fatigue.

To restore and maintain balance:

- Eat less sugar and smoked or cured meat.
- Eat more mucus-reducing foods, like garlic, seaweed, lemon, and chilies.
- Find space and time to process emotions.
- Stretch daily.

Dampness-Heat

People with this constitution tend to have oily skin, a bitter taste in the mouth, acne, and an aversion to humid weather.

To restore and maintain balance:

- Eat foods that move heat, like beans, basil, cucumber, and watermelon.
- Avoid fried food.
- Stay in a cool place during hot and humid times of year.
- Relieve stress with high-intensity exercise.

Qi Stagnation

People with this constitution struggle with stress, shallow breathing, and insomnia.

To restore and maintain balance:

- Eat more foods that clear stagnation, such as alliums, parsley, seaweed, radish, and kale.
- Breathe deeply before sleep and keep the bedroom dark and quiet.
- Engage in vigorous movement.
- Find activities that clear the mind.

Intrinsic Constitution

People with this constitution tend to have seasonal allergies, rashes and congestion, and difficulty transitioning between seasons.

To restore and maintain balance:

- Eat simply, focusing on animal foods and vegetables.
- Avoid spicy food.
- Keep pets outside.
- Enjoy gentle movement daily.

Note: These descriptions offer just an initial glimpse into the intricate world of TCM diagnostics and are not meant to replace the more informed assessment of a Chinese medicine practitioner. If you are curious to learn more, reach out to your local acupuncturist.

GRECO-ROMAN TRADITIONAL HEALING

The Greco-Roman healing tradition sees health as an interplay of four elements, four humors, and four temperaments.[3] The current Mediterranean way of seasonal eating and understanding its alignment with healing certain organ systems is rooted in healing systems from the Greek and Roman traditions. These traditions are have roots in Egyptian and Islamic systems of wellness, which in turn are influenced by Ayurveda and Chinese Medicine.

The Four Elements

This tradition holds that four elements comprise and influence all life: fire, air, water, and earth. These elements have qualities that apply both to the external environment and to our internal landscape: hot, dry, moist, and cold. Just as is the case for other traditional systems of healing, multiple qualities play a role in each element's actions. Air is hot and damp. Fire is hot and dry. Water is damp and cold. Earth is cold and dry.

The concept of something being hot is both about its temperature and about its energetic quality. Hot is describing the warmth of life as opposed to the chill of death. Therefore, the air element, which enlivens our being with breath, is seen as hot because the body requires heat to live.

Pneuma is our life force energy (like *qi* in Chinese medicine or *prana* in Ayurveda). Its name is the Greek word meaning "that which is breathed." In the Greco-Roman tradition, pneuma is a life-giving breath. The four elements influence pneuma in their own ways. Air adapts *pneuma* and represents spring and youth. Fire transforms *pneuma* and represents summer and childhood. Water receives *pneuma* and represents autumn and middle age. Earth condenses *pneuma* and represents winter and old age.

The Four Humors

The four humors explain how the body creates energy through metabolism of everything that it takes in through the environment (see plate 1 for a diagram). They move in a cyclical way. There is no beginning or end, just circular movement through nonlinear time. Day fades into night and night blends into day once again. The seasons wrap around each other and turn the wheel of life. The Greek medical writer Alcmaeon of Croton first described the four humors around 500 BCE. He identified them as blood, yellow bile, phlegm, and black bile. However, the humors likely originated in Egyptian or Mesopotamian healing systems long before his writing as a way to identify how human tendencies cycle with nature.

The word *humor* comes from the Latin *umor,* meaning moisture. As defined by Alcmaeon, the humors are the way in which humans manifest their life force energy, which is much like the sap, or lymph, that gives plants their life-giving moisture. In this system, blood is hot and moist. It aligns with the liver, air, and spring. Is this sounding familiar? Yellow bile is hot and dry. It corresponds with fire and summer. Phlegm is moist and cold. It aligns with autumn and water. Black bile is cold and dry. It aligns with winter and earth.

The Four Temperaments

The four temperaments—sanguine, choleric, phlegmatic, and melancholic—explain how the elements and humors manifest in the body and personality. The sanguine type of person relates to air and blood. Characteristics include sociability, enthusiasm, and a tendency to feel more impacted by stress than others. The choleric type connects with fire and yellow bile. Choleric types have a sharp mind and a great deal of ambition, and they tend to anger easily. The phlegmatic type relates to water and phlegm. Characteristics include being emotionally sensitive and aware as well as thoughtful and reserved. Melancholic types connect with earth and black bile. They are grounded when balanced and can tend toward wistfulness and depression. As we have seen in the personality/constitutional types described by Ayurveda and TCM, the Greco-Roman tradition holds that most of us have more than one predominant type, and these types can shift during different life stages.

The Mediterranean Way

In the tradition in which I was raised in northern Italy, food is medicine. We followed what is popularly called today the "Mediterranean Diet," which is founded in the Greco-Roman healing system. Key components include preparing fresh food with local, seasonally available ingredients and preserving the harvest. Growing up, we enjoyed soups, stews, rice, homemade egg pasta, chicory, barley beverages, and plenty of wild-crafted mushrooms and herbs. Including all the flavors and colors in each meal is considered essential to well-being. Plates are filled with colorful vegetables and whole grains, and olive oil (first cold press) and animal foods (meat, dairy, and so on) are considered condiments.

The Mediterranean way of eating has been touted as a strategy to reduce inflammation in our bodies and minds and promote longevity, and it's easy to see why. My family enjoyed Sunday meals with friends and relatives. Every dish was freshly made, warmed and finished in the final moments before serving. Everyone ate quietly, savoring each bite. Between courses, we talked. This way of eating is a way of life. It offers a model for learning to tune in to our daily practices with mindfulness and intention.

In the 1950s, physiologist Ancel Keys and his colleagues organized the Seven Countries Study to examine the theory that certain dietary practices contributed to longevity. Their study followed more than a thousand middle-aged men (women have not been the subject of studies until recent years) in the United States, Japan, Italy, Greece, the Netherlands, Finland, and what was then Yugoslavia. Data revealed that people whose eating centered around fruits and vegetables, grains, beans, and fish maintained vibrant health into old age. Researchers coined this way of eating the "Mediterranean diet," and it quickly became associated with wellness. Many more studies have since confirmed the health benefits of traditional Mediterranean food choices, showing that they may help improve quality of life into old age, support brain function and cardiovascular health, balance mood, and promote dental health.

Portion Guidelines

When I came to the States, I was astounded by the portions people ate. They were easily double what I had been accustomed to eating in Italy. In the Mediterranean, there is no such thing as an all-you-can-eat buffet. We stop eating before we are full and feel satisfied because we have taken the time to eat slowly and savor each bite.

I was confused by all the choices at every meal, even in my high school cafeteria. I wanted fewer options and ingredients I could recognize. I started inviting my new American friends to my house for dinner. We would cook together, taste ingredients before they went into the meal, and sit down to enjoy the results. I was struck by my friends commenting on how satisfied they felt even though we were eating less food than what was habitual for them.

When food is whole and simple, the flavors shine so that both the body and the soul are nourished. And though portion sizes are different for everyone, following portion guidelines can be helpful when trying to get a sense of how much food you truly need to thrive. Eating slowly and stopping before you feel too full is the key to determining the ideal portion sizes for you.

Constructing a Meal

Here are some general guidelines for healthy eating from the Mediterranean way of eating. As always, take into account your own unique needs, including those influenced by your heritage, before ascribing to any one way of eating.

- Whole grains can make up about a third of each meal. Whole grains include amaranth, buckwheat, millet, quinoa, rice, and wild rice.
- Vegetables typically make up about a third of each meal. Vegetables can be raw (in the summer), steamed, boiled, roasted, or sautéed.
- Proteins, such as fatty fish, pastured poultry, beans, and lentils, comprise the remaining one-third of each meal. Cook beans and

lentils without salt and with seaweed to improve their digestibility. Seaweed, such as kombu, contains specific amino acids that help break down the insoluble fiber in legumes before we eat them. It also contains digestive enzymes to optimize the body's breakdown and absorption of foods paired with seaweed.[4]

- Fats, such as olive oil, ghee, unsweetened yogurt, and aged cheese, are eaten as condiments. They contribute some of the nutrients necessary to break down the carbohydrates and proteins in the meal.

- Fruit, seeds, and nuts are considered part of dessert. Eat them about thirty minutes after a meal.

Health Benefits

Do you experience food- and/or stress-related inflammation? Do you ever notice occasional anxiety or depression, drowsiness after meals, gas, bloating, nausea, joint pain, scratchy throat, nasal congestion, and skin rash? These, among other signs, are messages from your body asking for support. It will be helpful to listen to them.

Stress, environmental toxins, reduced physical activity, and lack of nutrient-dense foods all contribute to inflammation in the body. Sustained inflammation can, over time, affect the joints, kidneys, heart, and intestines and lead to serious conditions such as heart disease, cancer, and Alzheimer's disease. For these reasons, reducing inflammation is crucial to maintaining wellness.

The Mediterranean way of eating is well respected for its capacity to help reduce inflammation and promote vibrancy into old age. It boosts physical and mental health, provides a steady supply of energy, and reduces the risk of age-related diseases by serving up healthy fats, fiber-rich fruits and veggies, lots of water, and limited amounts of animal protein.

While processed foods with lots of sugar and refined carbohydrates trigger inflammation, whole foods are rich in anti-inflammatory compounds. Olive oil, for example, contains oleocanthal, which has the same anti-inflammatory action as ibuprofen. Spices like turmeric, ginger, and rosemary keep inflammation in check in the gut, muscles, and brain. Oily fish and nuts are rich in minerals and fatty acids that reduce inflammation in the joints and heart. Mushrooms and green herbs such as parsley and cilantro reduce inflammation while boosting immunity.

The Truth about Olive Oil

Traditionally, people around the globe consider certain foods to be sacred. In my native Italy, it's olive oil. It is made from olives harvested at the end of October, which is a time considered by pagan traditions to be the start of a new year. Indeed, olive oil brings renewal as well as a host of health benefits.

Monounsaturated and liquid at room temperature, first cold-press olive oil has high levels of anti-inflammatory polyphenols, which reduce the risk of heart disease, help the body maintain a balanced cholesterol profile, and reduce the overgrowth of ulcer-inducing *Helicobacter pylori* bacteria in the intestines. It helps increase calcium and oxygen levels in the blood, thus also working to enhance memory function. Its antimicrobial volatile oils make it an excellent fat for maintaining a balanced gut microbiome free of potentially harmful pathogens.

Choose California organic olive oil or an imported olive oil that has the harvest date and acidity (less than 0.5 percent) labeled on the bottle.

The FDA does not regulate labeling on imported olive oil very stringently. This is why boutique olive oil stores exist. The oils sold in these stores have been tested by an independent laboratory that confirms the provenance of the oil and how it was processed. If you are buying imported olive oil, take time to research the source. Domestic oil labeling in the United States is highly regulated, which is why I recommend buying high-quality California oil if you do not have access to a trustworthy imported olive oil. It's important to make sure the oil is pressed rather than refined—processed with heat or alkali—so that the beneficial properties are maintained and negative properties aren't introduced. To learn more about olive oil sourcing and labeling, read Tom Mueller's book *Extra Virginity*.

We live in a world rich with whole foods. We need to reclaim our sovereign ability to choose them for our well-being. Our bodies are the best teachers of which foods provide healing and promote wellness. The more we listen, the more we can tune in and make the best food choices in any moment.

Recipes

The following recipes come from the Mediterranean tradition and call for anti-inflammatory unsaturated fats.

♠ Farinata Pizza

Farinata is a kind of pizza that originated in Genova, Italy. It is made primarily of chickpea flour, which is high in fiber and a plant-based protein. Farinata pizza is often offered during aperitivo, an Italian evening tradition where people gather to talk about the day while enjoying food and drinks.

For the dough:

> 2 cups chickpea flour
> ½ cup arrowroot flour
> 1 egg, beaten
> 3 tablespoons olive oil, plus a drizzle for coating the
>   dough and oiling the baking sheet
> 1½ cups warm water
> ¼ teaspoon sea salt
> 1 teaspoon dried rosemary
> 1 teaspoon dried oregano

For the topping:

> 1 cup cooked cannellini beans
> 1 cup basil
> 1 cup flat-leaf parsley
> ¼ cup olive oil
> Juice of 1 lemon
> 3 cloves garlic
> ¼ teaspoon salt

Preheat the oven to 400°F.

To prepare the dough, mix the ingredients together in a mixing bowl until a dough ball forms. Add more warm water if it feels a bit dry. Once the dough comes together in a slightly sticky ball, coat it with olive oil, place it back in the bowl, cover the bowl with a cloth, and set aside.

To prepare the topping, combine all the ingredients in a food processor and blend until a thick paste forms.

Oil a baking sheet with olive oil.

Press the dough into a thin layer on the oiled baking sheet. Do this with a loved one if you have the chance. Observe the difference between your fingerprints in the dough. Laugh when the dough bounces back and refuses to stretch. Strategize on who will hold down the corners of the dough and who will continue to press it to the edges. Know that the dough is doing what it must to remain flexible, elastic, alive.

Once you are satisfied with the shape and size of the dough, bake it for 15 minutes. Then remove the dough from the oven.

Spread the topping over the dough and return it to the oven to bake for 5 minutes more.

Remove from the oven and slice into squares. Enjoy in the company of beloveds while ruminating on the events of the day.

♠ Barley and Chicken with Mushrooms and Artichokes

The Italian word for barley is orzo. Orzo is valued in Italian cooking as a soothing, nourishing grain that is ideal for recovering from illness, strengthening children's muscles and bones, and supporting elders in the aging process. I grew up drinking orzo bimbo, a malted barley beverage that pairs well with a breakfast of soft-boiled eggs and fresh bread to dip into the yolks.

> 3 tablespoons olive oil
> 3 medium shallots, diced
> 1½ cups sliced cremini mushrooms
> 1 cup diced artichoke hearts

Salt and freshly ground black pepper

1 cup pearled barley

½ cup dry white wine

1 pound chicken tenders (hormone and antibiotic-free)

4 cups chicken or vegetable stock

1 cup grated Parmigiano Reggiano cheese (optional)

Preheat the oven to 350°F.

Heat the oil in an ovenproof pot over medium heat. Add the shallots, mushrooms, and artichokes, season well with salt and pepper, and cook, stirring occasionally, for about 5 minutes.

Reduce the heat to low and cook for 10 minutes more.

Add the barley. Increase the heat to medium and start stirring everything together. Stir until you hear the barley sizzle slightly.

Add the white wine and stir well to combine. Cook until all the wine has evaporated.

Reduce the heat to low. Nestle the chicken breasts on top of the barley and vegetables, and pour the stock over everything.

Cover, place in the oven, and bake for 30 minutes. If using the Parmigiano, scatter it over the chicken halfway through the baking process.

Remove from the oven and serve hot. You can finish it on the stovetop if the barley has not yet absorbed all the broth.

♠ Apricot Tahini Bread

This recipe originates in Turkey and has since graced the rest of the Mediterranean with its fragrant flavor. Apricots are high in vitamins A and C as well as anti-inflammatory antioxidants. Tahini is a paste of sesame seeds, which are higher in calcium than most dairy products and contain immune-boosting zinc.

1 cup chopped dried apricots

1½ cups boiling water

1½ cups almond flour

1½ cups oat flour

1 teaspoon baking powder

1 teaspoon baking soda

A pinch of salt

½ teaspoon ground cinnamon

¼ teaspoon ground cardamom

2 eggs, beaten

⅓ cup tahini

2 tablespoons olive oil, plus a bit for oiling the pan

1 tablespoon vinegar of choice

Place the chopped dried apricots in a bowl and pour the boiling water over them. Let them soak for 15 minutes.

Preheat the oven to 350°F.

Oil a loaf pan with olive oil and set aside.

Mix all the ingredients in the order listed.

Add the apricots and their soaking water. If the mixture is too crumbly, add a bit more water. It should have a doughlike consistency.

Bake for 30 minutes, or until a knife inserted into the center of the loaf comes out clean.

Let cool completely before slicing.

MANY WAYS OF HEALING

Though I focus on three traditional healing modalities—Ayurveda, traditional Chinese medicine, and the Greco-Roman healing system—I want to acknowledge that every indigenous group of people has its own specific healing tradition, and there are intersections among all of them. I will name a few, although by no means all.

One example of an unbroken system of healing that is upheld even today is that symbolized by the North American First Nations' medicine wheel. The wheel is a circular image that represents the circle of life, self-awareness, and knowledge. It is typically divided into four quadrants with four colors: red, yellow, black, and white. Each section represents a different state of being, season, sacred medicine, element, and stage of life. Different nations organize the colors and their meanings slightly differently.

Islam, a spiritual tradition practiced in much of the world, also sees healing as a cyclical process, with both health and illness affected by physical, metaphysical, spiritual, social, and environmental factors. Islamic philosophy considers illness to be a teaching about the ideal ways to maintain balance with the support of divine intervention. This system, known as traditional Arabic and Islamic medicine (TAIM) or Tibb Nabawi, the medicine of the Prophet Allah, is steeped in prophetic medicine from the sacred Quran. Its primary dietary teaching is fasting. Fasts are observed in tune with the cycles of the moon, planets, and seasons.[5] It is influenced by Persian and Mesopotamian medicine, which later became the Mediterranean system of healing. It also reflects aspects of Ayurveda and Chinese medicine.

Curanderismo, a holistic traditional healing system in Latin America, views disease as a state of being out of harmony with one's environment.[6] When curandero and patient work together to find balance, the connection between patient and the natural world is restored so the mind, body, and spirit regain health. Curanderos often use medicinal and psychedelic herbs to help restore harmony. This indigenous healing modality has ancient roots, having shifted to its modern form by incorporating elements of the Catholic colonial influence.

When I lived with the Diné people of the Diné Reservation, I learned about Diné Bahane, the Creation Story. The story is told to restore Są'a Naghái Bik'eh Hózhó, the Beauty Way. In the story, Talking God draws intersecting lines across the Earth, and nature springs from them. Similar lines can be seen in the intricate mandalas or sand paintings that Tibetan monks draw before erasing them to represent the ephemeral nature of reality. After my time with the Diné, I landed in a Tibetan settlement in Delhi and could not believe the similarities I saw and heard in spiritual practice and language.

The ancient connections between groups of people struck me so deeply that I started looking for intersections in the roots of my heritage—which led to this book. May you find the intersections in your own life and appreciate that, beyond our connection to indigenous people and lands, we are all indigenous to nature.

3

Organs, Seasons, and Systems

The Need for Food Rhythms

Dietary therapy should be the first step when one treats a disease. Only when this is unsuccessful should one try medicines.

SUN SIMIAO, TANG DYNASTY

Nourishment can take many forms. When we speak, breath and vibration combine to create sound, which feeds the spirit. Nourishment is not simply about getting the fuel needed to function. It is about satisfaction, enjoyment, grounding, as well as maintaining the health of the body's various organs and organ systems. The study of anatomy would like to chop us up into parts. However, we are intricate, somatic beings. What affects one system impacts all the others as well. Despite the current structure of our modern medical system, the body is not arranged according to medical specialties. Instead, both wellness and illness occur via intricate processes that involve all of the following systems working together, either in harmony or in dissonance:

- Energy (energy production, circadian rhythm, mitochondria)
- Assimilation (metabolism, nutrient absorption, gut microbiome, respiration)

- Biotransformation and elimination (detoxification, liver, large intestine)
- Defense and repair (immune, inflammation, infections, microbiota)
- Transport (cardiovascular, lymphatic system)
- Communication (endocrine/glandular system, neurotransmitters, brain)
- Structural integrity (from subcellular membranes to musculoskeletal structure)

The Institute for Functional Medicine refers to this concept as the functional medicine matrix, an inclusive framework of assessment and treatment that addresses root causes of disease, instead of symptoms.

There are many triggers for disease and many tools for restoring health. Food, however, is the foundation of wellness because we eat it every day. The food that is most digestible and health-promoting for each of us is part of our heritage and our genetic makeup. That said, the foods that are necessary for establishing and maintaining health are somewhat different for each of us depending both on our inherent makeup and on our life experiences. We can uncover our ideal foods through learning about ourselves on a deeper level.

What does a human being need to thrive? Because we are part of nature, our needs match those of the environment: air, water, protection from harsh elements, food, energy, and interrelationship. Carbon, water, nitrogen, oxygen—the same materials that comprise the Earth also make up our own blood and bones, our breath, and our brains. Our hair, skin, tears, and eventually entire bodies are all returned to the Earth, where they break down into these same materials. Since our bodies are literally made from Earth, we can use them directly to gain an understanding of the way Earth works.

Bill Mollison coined the term *permaculture* to mean a blending of permanent agriculture and permanent culture. This system involves the conscious design and maintenance of agriculturally productive ecosystems that have the diversity, stability, and resilience of natural ecosystems.

It calls for harmonious integration of landscape and people to create a regenerative system, one that nourishes itself to maintain homeostasis. A study of permaculture tells us that diversity alone is not enough. For any system to achieve resilience and health, meaningful connections must exist between the diverse elements of the system. This stability principle, as it's known, is as applicable to humans as it is to a garden.[1]

As a whole system, the body mirrors the principles of permaculture. A guild in permaculture is a combination of plants, animals, insects, and fungi that functions through collaboration. Similarly, the body is a blend of water, bones, organs, and bacteria working together. Each element contributes something valuable to the composition of the guild or body. For example, fungi recycle plants after they die and transform them into rich soil. If not for mushrooms, the Earth would be buried in debris and life would soon disappear. By the same token, the bacteria in our bodies digest food to produce waste. This waste nourishes the same soil that returns our food to us.

Anatomy and its concomitant medical disciplines would like to divide the body into its parts and examine them separately. The word *anatomy* comes from the Greek *tomia*, "to cut," and *ana*, "up." Anatomy is based in dissection, whereas somatics, the study of the body as a complex relationship between cells, comes from the Greek *soma*, "body." When we look at the body somatically instead of anatomically, we can see that we are complex beings, part of nature, and as much interconnected in ourselves as we are to our environment.

By aligning our bodies with the Earth's body, we can maintain the connections necessary to thrive and let our healing also become the Earth's healing. Since these systems are always changing, it is important to observe both seasonal changes and internal physical shifts so that we can respond to them. We can turn to centuries-old systems of using food as medicine as our guides to help us live with the flexibility that allows for resiliency.

Chinese medicine, Ayurveda, and the Mediterranean way, among other traditions, all ascribe to the principle of "as within, so without." They recognize the connections between body, mind, and spirit and the time, seasons, age, life circumstances, and interrelationships between these factors.

THE BODY CLOCK

Health is a constant process of dis-ease moving into ease and then back into dis-ease. Illness, pain, and food cravings are signals of the body's disharmony and offer insight on how to address root causes to restore homeostasis. Traditional nutritional philosophies are a tool to regain balance again and again. Ayurveda believes that all illness stems from *ama,* undigested food matter. Thus, cultivating *agni,* digestive fire, is crucial to health. By aligning with the seasons and supporting the relevant organs during seasonal transitions, we can maintain strong digestion and reduce ama. In the Ayurvedic tradition, fall and winter are vata (air) season; spring is kapha (earth) season; and summer is pitta (fire) season.

According to Ayurveda, every hour of the day is related to specific qualities. Different times of day have different strengths and weaknesses and can therefore help us determine both the best time to engage in certain activities and the most likely time for imbalances to occur. Knowing our internal body clock can help us align our daily activities to allow optimal functioning and therefore optimal health (see the following page for a diagram of the Ayurvedic body clock).

Another essential aspect of the Ayurvedic body clock is the relationship of the doshas to the time of day. Knowing the ebb and flow of the doshas can help us choose ideal times for certain activities. For example, it is best to eat our largest meal midday, as this is the time when pitta is strongest and we are likely to have the most digestive fire. The dinner meal should be much smaller and lighter, since kapha is high at this time. It's no surprise that Chinese medicine and the tenets of the Mediterranean way agree with these principles.

The doshas correlate not just to times of day but also to the seasons and emotions—and these factors also interconnect to each other. Ayurveda sees each year as being divided into eight seasons: early spring and late spring, early summer and late summer, early fall and late fall, and early winter and late winter.

AYURVEDIC BODY CLOCK CORRESPONDENCES

Dosha	Time of Day	Seasons	Temperature
Vata	2–6 a.m. and 2–6 p.m.	Early and late fall and early winter	cold and dry
Pitta	10 a.m.–2 p.m. and 10 p.m.–2 a.m.	Early and late summer and early fall	hot
Kapha	6–10 a.m. and 6–10 p.m.	Late winter and early and late spring	cool and wet

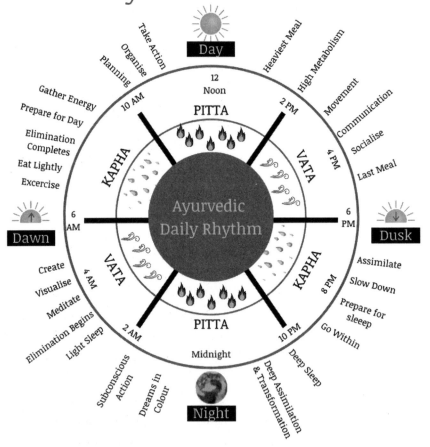

This is a depiction of the Ayurvedic body clock.

(Courtesy of Harmony Inspired Health, harmonyinspiredhealth.com.au.)

Do you ever get tired (kapha) after dinner and then get a second wind (pitta) if you stay up past bedtime? This is the body clock at work. During kapha (earthy) times of year, like late winter and early spring, we may find ourselves struggling during the kapha time windows (six to ten o'clock in the morning or evening) if we are kapha dominant. It may feel hard to get up in the morning or to wind down enough to go to sleep at night. Conversely, those with little kapha in their constitution will find it easier to wake up and go to bed during these times.

Chinese medicine offers parallels to the Ayurvedic body clock. There are slight differences, perhaps due to climatic differences between China and India. In Chinese medicine, the times of day correlate to elements and organs (see the following page for a diagram of the Chinese body clock). The fire element is repeated during the day because the heart is the center of shen, 神, the mind and consciousness. This heart-mind connection is foundational for all other body functions.

TUNING IN TO THE BODY CLOCK

Is there a time of day when you typically feel sluggish or tired? Is there a time when you are most vibrant? Notice which organs and energies these times match up with on the body clocks. Do you wake up consistently at a certain time of night? Make note of the correspondences for that time on the body clocks as well. These traditional systems offer tools for determining where we have hereditary weaknesses. They offer a pathway for understanding how we can work with imbalances instead of trying to eliminate them.

As an example, winter feels challenging for me; it always seems too cold and either too dry or damp. To find balance, I enjoy vigorous walks and skiing, hot soups, and warm baths. Instead of feeling frustrated that my body struggles in the colder months, I listen to its requests for support and try to honor them.

Is there an organ that tends to be a weak spot for you or an illness that recurs every year? After ten years of chronic intestinal parasites, I have digestive weakness, so I need to take extra care in the fall to support my large intestine. Before I understood this about myself, autumn was typically a time when my digestion would go haywire, and I would suffer for months before regaining balance. Now, I prepare for fall when summer begins to wane. I slow down, eat more simply, and let go of habits and foods that are not supportive.

CHINESE BODY CLOCK

Element	Time	Organ(s)	Flavor
Earth	7 to 11 a.m.	Stomach/spleen	Sweet
Fire	11 a.m. to 3p.m.	Heart/small intestine	Bitter
Water	3 to 7 p.m.	Bladder/kidney	Salty
Fire	7 to 11 p.m.	Pericardium / triple burner	Bitter
Wood	11 p.m. to 3 a.m.	Liver/gallbladder	Sour
Metal	3 to 7 a.m.	Lung/large intestine	Pungent

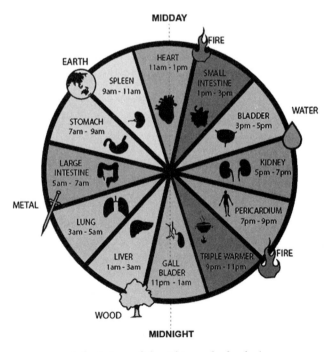

A depiction of the Chinese body clock.
(Courtesy of "Eating with the Chinese Bodyclock," by Purdy Rhodes for Quiescence Chinese Medicine.)

Make a list of any symptoms you notice in your body. Review the list of inflammation symptoms in chapter 9 and see which (if any) you experience. See whether you can correlate any of these symptoms to an organ. For example:

- Gas and bloating correspond to the large intestine and colon. To find balance, eat pungent food and slow down during autumn.
- Belching corresponds to the stomach. To find balance, enjoy cooked, warming orange foods and smaller portions in late summer.
- Joint pain and swelling correspond to liver inflammation. To find balance, follow a dietary simplification or cleanse in the spring.
- Heart palpitations and shortness of breath correspond to the heart. To find balance, enjoy bitter foods in the summer and take digestive bitters.

NOURISHMENT THROUGH THE SEASONS

We can nourish ourselves with more intention and alignment both by listening to the body's messages and by noticing the seasonal requirements and shifts. Winter requires warming foods cooked more slowly and time spent stretching and warming the body after being outside. The shift into spring calls for a simplified version of eating to support the organs in a process of renewal and expansion, which is reflected in the eventual blossoming of nature.

The Five Transformations

Because traditional Chinese medicine identifies five seasons throughout the year, the cycle of life and health is known as the five transformations: Spring becomes summer, summer becomes late summer, late summer becomes autumn, autumn becomes winter, and winter becomes spring, and the cycle regenerates.

Spring focuses on the wood element (sap rising in the trees), the sour flavor (dandelion greens, watercress, citrus), and cleansing the liver and gallbladder. Emotional tendencies are anger and patience.

Summer welcomes the fire element (circulation and energy), the bitter flavor (salad), and supporting the small intestine and heart. Summer's emotions are excitement and tranquility.

Late summer, known in Chinese medicine as the "great interchange of all seasons," is crucial for maintaining health all year round. It is focused on the earth element (digestion, immunity), the sweet flavor (winter squash, apples), and the spleen and stomach. Emotions are suspicion and compassion.

Autumn heralds the metal element (sticks and stones) and the pungent flavor (alliums and turnips) and calls for healing the lungs and large intestine. Autumn is for letting go of mental and emotional states that do not serve us.

Winter brings forth the water element (staying hydrated) and the salty flavor (maintaining water balance) and highlights the importance of caring for the bladder and kidneys. Fear and the will arise in winter.

Seasonal Energies and Mediterranean Eating

In the Greco-Roman system, foods, just like the four elements, have an energetic quality or thermal nature: They are warming, cooling, moist, or dry. A food's thermal nature can be impacted by cooking or adding spices, but its inherent qualities, just as with the human constitution, will not change.

These energetics carry over into determining which foods are appropriate during different seasons.

Spring is a time for bitter green foods, the first to sprout after a long winter: dandelion greens, watercress, leeks, peas, perennial herbs (rosemary, lavender, thyme, parsley). It is a good time for liver cleansing.

Summer is for sweet and spicy foods to support the circulatory and lymphatic systems: artichokes, red peppers, tomatoes, basil, garlic, apricots, berries, barley, buckwheat, oats, rye, wheat. Summer calls us outside to move and sweat.

Autumn celebrates the abundance of the harvest to support strong immunity and digestion all winter long: apples, pears, beets, carrots, mushrooms, olives, potatoes, winter squash. It's a good time for healing the gut.

Winter is a time for enjoying storage crops and the last offerings from the garden: cabbage, cauliflower, leeks, and parsnips. It lends an opportunity to rest and restore the nervous system.

NOURISHMENT THROUGH THE FIVE FLAVORS

In traditional Chinese medicine, as is true in Ayurveda, the Greco-Roman system, and most other traditional healing modalities, each organ system corresponds with and is nourished by a particular flavor.

Sweetness tends to be a predominant flavor in meals. Most grains, vegetables, and fruits represent the sweet flavor and the earth element, which influence the stomach and pancreas. When consumed with mindfulness, this flavor strengthens the body and improves mood. Too much sugar leads to excessive mucus and stagnation.

The sour flavor and the wood element influence the liver and gallbladder. Sour foods include vinegar, chicken, lemon, and tomatoes. Sourness has an astringent and consolidating effect in the body, which can control diarrhea and excess perspiration or help focus a scattered mind.

The salty flavor and the water element affect the kidneys and bladder. The excessive use of salt in most processed food is a cause of many illnesses. Salt in the small amounts found in seaweed moistens dryness, counteracts toxins, and calms the nerves. In excess, it is a purgative and can harm the kidneys.

The pungent or spicy flavor represents the metal element and addresses the lungs and large intestine. It can stimulate circulation. Pungent herbs like mint or garlic can be used to break up the mucus of a cold, and pungent spices like ginger can help soothe a stomachache.

The bitter flavor corresponds to the fire element and the heart. Bitterness removes heat and toxins, and bitter herbs like dandelion and echinacea work to detoxify the organs. Dark chocolate is bitter and in modest amounts is healing.

Ayurveda adds a sixth taste: astringent. Foods from the amaranth family (amaranth, beets, chard, quinoa, spinach) and citrus reflect this quality. The astringent flavor can help counteract mucus buildup or sluggish bowels.

EATING TO ALIGN WITH THE SEASONS

When we eat seasonally, we minimize the impact of stress because we are harmonizing our internal self with the external environment that surrounds and supports us. This intersection helps guide our practice of integrating food as medicine in our lives.

To align with each season, we can use meal plans from Chinese medicine while taking into account our Ayurvedic constitution and the principles of the Mediterranean way of eating.

Spring Meal Plan

Spring features fresh green foods as well as sour flavor to harmonize the liver. I love making a special spring feast of millet congee, lentil casserole, walnut pâté, and maple gingerbread. You can also include a side of sauerkraut.

🍐 Millet Congee

Congee is a grain dish indigenous to Asia. It is cooked for such a long time that the grain dissolves into a thick porridge. It is incredibly easy to digest and served to people who are healing from illness as well as children and elders. Millet is a gluten-free, mineral-rich whole grain. Chinese medicine considers it the "queen of grains" because its ratio of fat, protein, and carbohydrates is so well balanced.

Cultivated in central Asia and West Africa for thousands of years, millet is a small-seeded cereal in the Poaceae family, the largest grass family, which gains its name from the Greek poa, "grass." This family includes all grasses grown for their edible seeds, such as rice, wheat, rye, oats, and corn. Although many of these cereals have become annual crops, researchers like those at the Kansas-based Land Institute are working to develop an agricultural system of perennial cereal grasses "with a yield similar to that from annual crops."[2]

1 cup millet

4 cups vegetable broth

½-inch piece fresh ginger, grated

1 carrot, grated

2 tablespoons sesame oil

Rinse the millet under running water and drain well in a strainer.

Place all the ingredients in a stock pot. Heat until the mixture is just off the boil. Then reduce the heat to low, cover, and cook for 30 minutes.

Stir the congee every 5 minutes or so to help it thicken and to keep it from sticking to the bottom of the pot.

Ladle the congee into a bowl and enjoy as part of your spring feast. You might also enjoy the congee with a fried egg or cooked beans on top for breakfast.

Casserole of Lentils and Mustard Greens

1 cup dry red lentils

5 cups vegetable broth

¼ cup olive oil, plus a bit for oiling the pie plate

2 cloves garlic, minced

½ teaspoon salt

½ teaspoon freshly ground black pepper

1 bunch fresh mustard greens

½ teaspoon ground coriander

½ teaspoon ground cumin

Juice of ½ lemon

2 tablespoons stone-ground mustard (no sugar added)

Rinse and drain the lentils. Combine the lentils and broth in a stock pot over high heat. Bring to a boil, then reduce the heat to medium. Skim off any foam (the foam contains the constituents that can cause flatulence). Cook with the lid slightly askew until the lentils are creamy and have absorbed most of the liquid. This

will take about 15 minutes. Stir occasionally to make sure they
do not stick to the pot. Do not add salt.

Heat the oil in a skillet. Add the minced garlic, then reduce
the heat to low. Add the salt and pepper and simmer for a
couple of minutes.

Add the mustard greens. Smell the pungent fragrance that
arises and then dissipates as the greens cook. Simmer for
10 minutes, or until most of the liquid has cooked out of the
vegetables. Add a splash of water if the greens and garlic are
sticking to the bottom of the skillet.

Meanwhile, preheat the oven to 375°F. Grease a pie plate
with olive oil.

Mix the cooked greens with the cooked lentils, coriander,
cumin, mustard, and lemon juice.

Pour the lentil-vegetable mixture into the oiled pie plate and
bake for 40 minutes.

🍐 Walnut Pâté

> 1 yellow onion, chopped
> 4 tablespoons olive oil
> Salt and freshly ground black pepper
> Splash of lemon juice
> ½ cup walnut halves/pieces

Gently warm 1 tablespoon of oil in a skillet. Add the chopped
onions and season with salt and pepper. Sauté for 10 minutes
over low heat, stirring occasionally to make sure the onions
don't stick to the bottom of the skillet. You can add a bit of
water if they are sticking. Add a splash of lemon juice and turn
off the heat.

While the onions are cooking, place the walnuts in a dry
skillet over medium heat. Toast, tossing often with a spatula,
until they are lightly browned, about 3 minutes.

Once onions and walnuts are cooked, place them in a food processor and add the remaining 3 tablespoons olive oil. You can also place all ingredients in a deep bowl and blend with an immersion blender.

Blend at the highest speed for 2 minutes. Taste for salt.

This pâté keeps in the fridge for 5 days.

🍐 Maple Gingerbread

1½ cups almond flour

½ cup arrowroot flour

½ teaspoon baking powder

½ teaspoon baking soda

¼ teaspoon salt

½ teaspoon ground cinnamon

½ teaspoon ground ginger

⅛ teaspoon ground cloves

¼ teaspoon ground nutmeg

⅓ cup maple syrup

2 eggs, beaten

¼ cup coconut oil, melted, plus extra for greasing the baking dish

½ cup unsweetened applesauce

¼ cup hot water

2 teaspoons fresh lemon juice

Zest of 1 lemon

Preheat the oven to 350°F.

Grease a baking dish with coconut oil. I use either an 8 x 8-inch dish or a loaf pan.

Mix all the ingredients together in the order listed. Spread evenly in the baking dish. Bake for 30 minutes, or until a knife inserted into the center comes out clean.

Let cool for at least 15 minutes before slicing.

Summer Meal Plan

Summer features more fresh vegetables, cooling foods, and the bitter flavor to harmonize the stomach. The recipes here—quinoa burgers, parsley cilantro gremolata, eggs poached in beet greens, and strawberry shortcake—come together as a wonderful meal to make with a group because everyone can participate.

Quinoa Burgers

> Olive oil, for greasing the baking sheet
> 1½ cups cooked quinoa
> 1 cup shredded zucchini
> ¼ cup ground flaxseed
> 2 heaping spoonfuls tahini
> 1 tablespoon olive oil
> 1 teaspoon mustard of choice
> ¼ teaspoon salt
> ½ teaspoon ground coriander
> ½ teaspoon ground cumin
> ½ cup plant milk

Preheat the oven to 375°F. Grease a baking sheet with olive oil.

Combine all the other ingredients in a mixing bowl. Stir until thoroughly blended.

Shape patties of any size by rolling dough into a ball with your hands and flattening it onto the baking sheet.

Bake for 15 minutes, flip with a spatula, bake for 15 more minutes, and enjoy.

Parsley Cilantro Gremolata

The Italian word gremolata comes from the dialect of Milan and essentially means "to granulate." Gremolata is traditionally made with a mortar and pestle. Although this is a recipe from the Mediterranean summer tradition, it pairs perfectly with Chinese medicine's recommendations.

3 tablespoons olive oil

¼ cup chopped scallions (optional)

¼ teaspoon salt

½ tablespoon lemon juice

I bunch fresh flat-leaf parsley, roughly chopped

I bunch fresh cilantro, roughly chopped

Combine all the ingredients in a blender and blend at the highest speed for 2 minutes. Enjoy at will. Try topping your quinoa burgers with a spoonful or two.

🍆 Eggs Poached in Beet Greens

I bunch tender young beet greens or Swiss chard (about
  2 packed cups)

Salt and freshly ground black pepper

A few garlic cloves

A sprinkle of sesame seeds (optional)

4 eggs

Chopped fresh basil

Rinse the greens, then place them in a wide skillet with ½ inch of water. Cover, bring to a boil, then reduce the heat to a simmer.

Season the greens with salt and pepper. Crush a few garlic cloves over the greens, and sprinkle them with sesame seeds if you like.

Create four shallow indentations in the greens, then crack the eggs into them. Place the lid on the skillet and angle it to leave enough of an opening for steam to escape.

Slowly poach the eggs over low heat for 5 to 6 minutes for soft yolks (8 to 9 minutes for hard yolks).

Meanwhile, chop a handful of basil. Sprinkle the basil over the poaching eggs and steam briefly.

Remove each egg from the skillet with a bit of greens and place on plates alongside quinoa burgers topped with gremolata.

🫐 Strawberry Shortcake

For the strawberries:

> 1½ pounds strawberries, stemmed and quartered
>
> 2 tablespoons raw honey
>
> 1 teaspoon fresh lemon juice
>
> ¼ teaspoon ground cinnamon

For the shortcake:

> 1 cup cornmeal
>
> 1 cup oat flour
>
> ¼ cup arrowroot flour
>
> ½ teaspoon baking powder
>
> ½ teaspoon baking soda
>
> A pinch of salt
>
> ¼ teaspoon ground cardamom
>
> ¼ teaspoon ground cinnamon
>
> ⅛ teaspoon ground nutmeg
>
> ¼ cup coconut oil, plus a bit for oiling the baking sheet
>
> Juice of ½ lemon
>
> 2 tablespoons maple syrup
>
> 1 teaspoon vanilla extract
>
> Whipped Coconut Cream (page 73), for topping
> (optional)

Prepare the strawberries: Combine the berries with the honey, lemon juice, and cinnamon. Toss gently and set aside.

Preheat the oven to 375°F. Oil a baking sheet with bit of coconut oil or olive oil.

Make the shortcake: Combine the cornmeal, oat flour, arrowroot flour, baking powder, baking soda, salt, cardamom, cinnamon, and nutmeg in large bowl and whisk together.

Cut in the coconut oil in small pieces and toss well, so that little pea-sized pearls of coconut oil are coated in the flour mixture.

Then add the lemon juice, maple syrup, and vanilla and mix

to incorporate. If the dough seems too dry, add a few spoonfuls of cold water.

Shape the dough into balls, and flatten them slightly into hockey puck shapes on the baking sheet.

Bake for 15 minutes, or until a toothpick inserted into the center comes out clean.

Top with the strawberries and whipped coconut cream, if you like.

Whipped Coconut Cream

    1 cup coconut milk
    1 teaspoon vanilla extract
    2 tablespoons raw honey
    2 tablespoons coconut butter
    Zest of 1 lemon

Whip all the ingredients together with an immersion blender or in a food processor.

Autumn Meal Plan

Autumn features sweeter, cooked foods like root vegetables and winter squash as well as the pungent flavor to harmonize the lungs and large intestine. This is a time for cooking foods more slowly and for longer periods of time. I return to the kitchen as my hearth and my anchor with this meal: immune-boosting soup, brown rice pilaf, and squash pie.

Immune-Boosting Soup

Start heating a pot of cold water on the stovetop.

Add:

    3 chicken legs, beef with bones, lamb shanks, or other
        meat on the bone (optional)
    A handful of chopped astragalus root, for immune support
    A handful of fresh or dried shiitake or maitake mushrooms
    2-inch piece of kombu seaweed, rinsed

½ teaspoon salt

2 carrots, chopped into quarters

2 stalks celery, chopped in half

1 onion, whole, with peel removed

1 head garlic, whole, with outer flaky part of the peel
removed

Cover the pot and bring to a boil, then lower the heat and simmer
for 1 to 2 hours, until any meat falls off the bones.

Remove the bones, herbs, any dried mushrooms, and roots
from the soup.

Now, you can add other vegetables and herbs, such as:

Aromatic vegetables, like leeks, mustard greens, parsnips,
and turnips—these reduce congestion

Orange vegetables, like carrots, sweet potatoes, and
winter squash—these are rich in carotenoids, which
support immunity and respiratory health

Herbs and spices, like black pepper, oregano, and
thyme—these are antimicrobial and reduce the risk of
contracting an infection

Simmer the soup until everything is tender, then add more
garlic and ginger if you like. Taste for salt.

🍐 Rice and Mushroom Pilaf

1 cup brown rice

2 cups vegetable or chicken broth

1 tablespoon coconut oil

1 large yellow onion, chopped

3 stalks celery, chopped

8 ounces shiitake mushrooms, sliced

2 cloves garlic, minced

1 teaspoon oregano

1 teaspoon sage

1 teaspoon thyme

½ teaspoon salt

½ cup chopped pecans or walnuts

Place the rice and vegetable broth in a large saucepan, bring the mixture to a boil, then lower the heat and simmer, covered, for 35 to 40 minutes, until the broth is completely absorbed.

While the rice is cooking, melt the coconut oil in a large Dutch oven over medium heat. Add the onion and celery and sauté until tender, about 8 minutes. Add the mushrooms, garlic, oregano, sage, thyme, and salt and sauté another 8 to 10 minutes, until the mushrooms are tender.

Combine the cooked rice with the mushroom mixture and stir in the pecans or walnuts. Adjust any seasoning to taste and serve warm.

🍐 Soothing Squash Pie

For the filling:

I winter squash

2 tablespoons maple syrup

3 eggs, beaten

2 tablespoons flaxseed meal

½ teaspoon ground cinnamon

¼ teaspoon ground allspice

¼ teaspoon ground nutmeg

A pinch of salt

For the crust:

Sunflower oil, for oiling the pie plate

I cup pecan or almond flour

¼ cup flaxseed meal

¼ cup coconut oil

½ cup plant milk

¼ teaspoon ground cinnamon

¼ teaspoon ground ginger

A pinch of salt

I egg, beaten

Preheat the oven to 400 degrees F.

Make the filling: Bake the whole squash for 1 hour, or until knife tender. Remove from the oven, cut open, scoop out the seeds, and allow to cool. Once cooled, scoop out flesh; you should have about 3 cups. Place in a food processor with all the other filling ingredients. Blend well.

As squash bakes, prepare the crust: Oil a 9-inch pie plate with sunflower oil. Mix all the other ingredients together. Press the crust into the bottom of the pie plate.

Once your filling is well blended, smooth it over the crust.

Bake at 400°F for 15 minutes, then lower the oven heat to 350°F and bake for another 25 minutes.

Winter Meal Plan

Winter is a time to replenish minerals in our tissues and harness the flow of the water that comprises so much of our bodies. The salty flavor is the tool to harmonize the kidneys and hardworking adrenal glands. This winter meal of black bean stew, buckwheat pancakes, sesame seaweed salad, and pear cake feels both restorative and energizing during those long nights.

🍐 Black Bean Stew

3 tablespoons coconut oil

1 onion, chopped

3 cups chicken broth

½ teaspoon ground coriander

½ teaspoon ground cumin

¼ teaspoon ground cinnamon

¼ teaspoon ground fenugreek

¼ teaspoon freshly ground black pepper

¼ teaspoon salt

1 large sweet potato (about 1 pound), peeled and cut into ½-inch pieces

1-inch piece of kombu or wakame seaweed, chopped with scissors

1 tablespoon fresh lemon juice

1 cup cooked black beans

Heat the olive oil in a soup pot over medium heat until hot. Add the onion and sauté briefly.

Stir in ⅓ cup of the broth and cook for 5 minutes.

Stir in the coriander, cumin, cinnamon, fenugreek, pepper, and salt. Cook 1 minute, stirring. Then add the remaining 2⅔ cups of the broth, along with the sweet potato, seaweed, and lemon juice.

Bring to a boil over medium-high heat. Reduce the heat to low, cover, and simmer for about 20 minutes, or until the sweet potato is tender.

Add the black beans, let simmer until the beans are warmed through, and serve.

Easy Beans

This technique works well for cooking any kind of dried bean.

Soak 1 cup dried beans in 4 cups cold water overnight.

The next morning, drain off the water and put the beans in a stock pot with 4 cups water. Bring to a boil, then reduce the heat to hold a simmer. Skim off any foam that rises to the top. Let the beans cook until tender. This usually takes about 25 minutes. Chickpeas will take 45 minutes.

Drain and rinse the beans. Set them aside in the refrigerator and add them to soup or sauté them with olive oil, salt, and cumin to savor as a side dish. You can store the beans in the refrigerator for up to five days or freeze them for up to a month.

Buckwheat Pancakes

¼ cup olive oil, plus a bit for oiling the pan

2 cups buckwheat flour

½ teaspoon salt

3½ cups water

Combine all the ingredients and mix well.

Heat a skillet (preferably cast iron) and drizzle in a little olive oil. Pick up the skillet by the handle and rotate it until the bottom is coated with oil.

Reduce the heat to low and ladle a scoop of batter into the skillet. Let the batter sit until bubbles form on top, then flip the pancake and let it cook 2 to 3 minutes more.

Repeat this process with the remaining batter. You may need to oil the skillet again if it is stainless steel. The initial oiling will suffice for cast iron.

Sesame Seaweed Salad

> 2 cups chopped dried seaweed (I like equal parts dulse and kombu)
> 1 tablespoon tamari
> 1 teaspoon maple syrup
> 1 tablespoon apple cider vinegar
> 1 tablespoon toasted sesame oil
> 3 tablespoons sesame seeds

Rinse your seaweed in cold water and soak in more cold water for 15 minutes. Mix together the rest of the ingredients to make the dressing. Toss the dressing with the seaweed. Let marinate for 15 to 30 minutes before eating.

Store any leftovers in the refrigerator, where they will keep for up to 1 week.

Pear Cake

> 2 firm pears
> ¾ cup maple syrup
> 1 cup brown rice flour
> 1 cup oat flour
> ½ cup buckwheat flour
> ½ teaspoon baking soda

½ teaspoon baking powder

½ teaspoon ground cinnamon

¼ teaspoon ground cardamom

¼ teaspoon ground nutmeg

¼ teaspoon salt

3 eggs, beaten

¼ cup olive oil, plus a bit for oiling the skillet

2 tablespoons apple cider vinegar

I cup oat milk

Preheat the oven to 350°F.

Oil a 9-inch cast iron skillet with olive oil.

Slice the pears and arrange them on the bottom of the skillet. Drizzle ¼ cup of the maple syrup over the pears and simmer on the stovetop for 5 minutes. Then remove the skillet from the heat.

Meanwhile, mix the rest of the ingredients together in the order listed to make the cake batter.

Note: If you would like to make your own fresh flours, you can grind brown rice, oats, and buckwheat separately in an espresso bean grinder. You can also substitute 2 cups almond flour and I cup arrowroot flour for a grain-free version of this cake.

Pour the batter over the pears. Bake for 45 minutes, or until a toothpick inserted into the center of the cake comes out clean.

Let the cake cool for 20 minutes. Then run a knife around its edge to separate it from the skillet. Place a plate on top of the skillet. Holding the plate with one hand and the skillet handle with the other, flip the cake out onto the plate.

Note: You can also make this cake with a cake pan. If you do, then at the end, after the cake comes out of the oven, place the plate on top of it, hold the pan and the plate with both hands, and flip. If the cake doesn't drop immediately, be patient. Set it down and tap on the bottom of the pan until you hear it loosen and thud down onto the plate.

4

Toward Intuitive Eating

Nourishment beyond Food

Health is not a state we owe the world. We are not less valuable, worthy, or lovable because we are not healthy. Lastly, there is no standard of health that is achievable for all bodies.

SONYA RENEE TAYLOR

When my parasitic infection first flared up and became chronic, I was doing things I loved: playing music, writing poetry, organizing, and feeding people in my role as kitchen manager for a worker-owned café I had founded with friends a year earlier. I was also working late nights and early mornings. Coffee and day-old muffins were my primary sources of nourishment. As my gut began burning and my anxiety began escalating, I had to give up working my favorite Saturday-night shift. I had to stop playing drums because I was in too much pain.

I hired a co-manager for the café kitchen, who was both incredibly talented and had the same questions I had about the ingredients we were using. They were all organic, but we had made some compromises, using sugar instead of maple syrup and eggs from cage-free chickens instead of pastured ones because these foods were (and still are) more affordable. The frustration of not being able to feed people the way

I wanted to, the stress of running a nascent business, the exhausting schedule, and my poor food choices triggered the flare-up.

Unfortunately, it is very human to push ourselves well beyond our limits before realizing that we have gone too far. As a pitta (fire) type, I tend to push my boundaries. The crash that ensued this time around was one that would inform the rest of my life to date.

I eventually had to sell my share of the café. Though my friends supported me, they did not understand why I had to step away. At that time, neither did I. I felt like I was dying but did not know why. I presented like a healthy person on the surface because I was in my early twenties. It was not until a year after I stepped away from our business that I discovered I had chronic intestinal parasites.

Through my healing journey, I started to understand that the energy we put into growing, harvesting, and cooking food is reflected in how we feel when we eat it. I realized why, when I was growing up, my family would pause to say a prayer before meals: It calms the enteric nervous system in the gut, thereby preparing us for proper digestion. I learned that the healing power of food comes both from what we eat and from how we eat it. Food is not just fuel, and eating is not just another task to check off the list. The sacred act of preparing and savoring food is the foundation for who we are.

WHAT IS MINDFUL EATING?

Mindful eating is a practice handed down through many traditions. From praying or offering gratitude before a meal to lighting a candle at dinner or eating in silence, this practice involves paying full attention to the experience of eating and drinking, both inside and outside the body. With mindful eating, the mind is full of the experience of eating. Thoughts about the past or future fade away. Attention is full of the colors, smells, textures, flavors, and sounds of food. Engaging deeply with the act of enjoying a meal both enhances the experience of the meal and soothes the nervous system, thus reducing stress.

When the mind wanders to what just happened or what will happen next, a mindful eater brings it back to the food without judgment. The mind often leans into distraction or multitasking while we are eating, and we end up reading, engaging with a screen, or some other mind-busying task. This is a normal tendency. They key is to notice when it's happening and to choose either to stop eating and follow the distraction or to return to the act of eating. In bringing our attention to the present moment, there is freedom, a joyful experience that we can attain every time we eat.

Eating with full presence takes practice. These suggestions can support a mindful eating routine.

First, Breathe

Breath is our first source of nourishment. Deep breathing relaxes not only the central nervous system (CNS) but also the enteric nervous system (ENS). The ENS resides in our intestines and is responsible for producing the neurotransmitters that release most of our stress hormones. When the gut remains at ease over time, anxiety and depression are alleviated. Taking a deep breath before eating is a simple way to not only ease stress but also to support our digestion and center our mind on the food in front of us.

Practice Affirmations

Honor your food by starting meals with an affirmation. Here are some examples:

> *This food is a gift from nature.*
> *May everyone have access to plenty of nourishing food.*
> *May this food help me be healthy, strong, and peaceful.*

Practice Silence

Try to eat one meal a week in silence so that you can be fully immersed in the experience of eating. Engage all the senses. As you serve and eat your meal, notice the sounds, colors, smells, and textures as well as your mind's response to them, not just the taste. When you put the first bite of food in your mouth, pause briefly before chewing and notice its taste as if it were the first time you had ever tasted it. With more practice in engaging all the senses, you may notice that your tastes change, increasing your enjoyment of food.

Practice Moderation

Moderation is an essential component of mindful eating. Making a conscious choice to eat smaller portions allows stretch receptors in the stomach and the satiety hormone, leptin, to send proper fullness cues to the brain. Choose a favorite small plate or bowl with which to eat meals and commit to filling it only once. If you truly feel hungry twenty minutes after eating a meal, have a second portion. Chinese medicine recommends we eat only until we are about 80 percent full and to avoid overfilling the stomach, which can weaken digestion.

Eat Slowly

Eating slowly creates space for relaxation and savoring the flavors of a meal. It also strengthens digestion; when the nervous system is in its "rest and digest" parasympathetic mode, we assimilate and use our food for energy far more effectively than when we eat on the run or while stressed.

One way to slow down is to put down your utensils between bites or to try noticing your breath while you are eating. Another is to eat smaller bites and chew each one well.

Don't Skip Meals

Try not to miss a meal. When we miss a meal, it can feel more challenging to make thoughtful choices later in the day. The body appreciates consistency, so plan a meal rhythm and try to stick to it. If you tend to skip breakfast because you don't feel hungry first thing in the morning, try eating your last meal of the day at 5 p.m. and then see how you feel the next morning.

Develop Ritual

Set aside five to ten minutes to enjoy each meal so that food and eating become a source of pleasure in your days. Light a candle. Lay out your utensils. Sit down to eat. If you have small children, let them sing a song of their own creation as you as you prepare to eat.

Create a small altar with a candle or incense. It can be a portable altar if you work on the move. Set it up for yourself before you eat, and use the element of fire to purify your energy. Though it can be hard to implement at first, many people find this practice supportive for the body, mind, and spirit. It can help dissolve mental constructs that feel like problems but are simply obstacles on the path to self-knowledge.

It can take time to become more focused on the practice of eating mindfully. Eventually, over time, you will start to notice that healthy eating is just as much about what you eat as it is about how you eat. Eating this way creates space to relax during the day and can help make meals feel like a gift rather than a stressor. Your life will feel more full.

STRESS MANAGEMENT

I would never have imagined that stress would play such a profound role in my journey to heal from chronic infection. But as it turns out, the transformation I experienced thanks to a silent meditation retreat at the Insight Meditation Society (IMS) was astounding. This beautiful retreat center in Massachusetts was created by meditators—including Jack Kornfield and Sharon Salzberg once they returned from their extensive Buddhist meditation studies in Asia—so that Westerners could benefit from the teachings.

A dear friend who practiced meditation had been encouraging me to attend a retreat with her. For a long time, I hesitated. I had been housebound for almost two years with chronic illness and debilitating pain. I cooked all my own food and was terrified to go anywhere outside my comfort zone because of the risk of worsening my symptoms. However, I had started having panic attacks and realized that something in my life needed to shift. After a year of consideration, I decided to attend a retreat with her. She talked me through exactly what it would be like and assured me that all the food prepared in the retreat center's kitchen was wholesome and nourishing. I also learned that the center had a fridge where attendees could store food they had brought with them.

I cooked and froze meals for the entire week away. I felt safer and more prepared for the adventure. I walked into IMS with my two coolers and a backpack full of clothes. I wore all the clothes, but I did not eat any of the food. After just one forty-minute session of silent meditation, I could feel my nervous system relaxing and my gut settling down. I then went into the dining hall and served myself breakfast. The staff had made plain oatmeal and offered many toppings in separate containers. It was simple, clear, and delicious. My enteric nervous system felt safe and communicated that feeling to my brain. My brain responded that it also felt calm thanks to the meditation and deep breathing.

I went through that retreat having a tremendous reduction in symptoms. Prior to attending, I had daily headaches that started every afternoon. I could eat only two or three bites of food before feeling so terribly full that I had to rest. I had chronic intestinal cramping, gas, bloating, constipation, and diarrhea, experienced insomnia for three hours most nights, and had started to develop a tremor in my left hand. But during the retreat, I did not experience any of those symptoms. Zero. When I returned home, some symptoms resurfaced, but only occasionally.

I realized that stress played a huge role in my illness, and that breathwork, mindfulness, and other stress management techniques could help. I knew it was time for change.

Stress in the Body

Stress is a physical expression of our sympathetic nervous system's survival mechanism. The word *stress* comes from the Latin *strictus,* "drawn tight." A threatening situation triggers a stress response, which prepares us to either face or run from danger. This reaction helps us survive immediate danger. However, the sympathetic response is also triggered by situations that are emotionally or psychologically stressful, and when stress builds up in our system, it can lead to inflammation and illness.

There are two main types of stress: acute and chronic. Acute stress, also known as the "fight or flight" response, is the body's sympathetic nervous system responding to a situation that it perceives as a crisis. During an acute stress response, the adrenal glands, located on top of each kidney, release a variety of hormones. Blood glucose rises, blood pressure increases, and digestion stops.

Chronic stress occurs when continuous acute stress keeps the body on alert. The ongoing stress response causes the hypothalamus and pituitary gland in the brain to produce hormones that stimulate the adrenal glands to release cortisol, one of the hormones associated with our wake-sleep cycle. Normally cortisol levels are highest in the morning, to help us wake up, and lowest at night, to help us sleep. When chronic stress stimulates cortisol production, the daily cycle of cortisol levels is disrupted, resulting in insomnia, headaches, and mood imbalances.

Chronic stress has many other serious negative impacts on our overall wellness as well—entire books have been written on the subject.

Stress Management Techniques

Practicing stress management techniques can help minimize the impact of stress. Though we'll focus here on just two techniques—eating and breathwork—there are many others. One of the best-studied techniques is exercise; sometimes just taking a short walk after experiencing emotional stress is enough to release the tension.

What We Eat

Every food we eat impacts our stress response. Refined cane sugar and high-fructose corn syrup, for example, are highly addictive nonfoods that contribute to chronic stress. It is challenging to metabolize these foods because they are stripped of the fiber and protein we need to digest them properly. They also have a high glycemic index, causing a quick rise in blood glucose followed by an immediate crash, which simply leads the body to crave more of them to get the fleeting high again.

Instead of getting stuck on the blood glucose roller coaster, try to eat foods that stabilize blood sugar and soothe the nervous system, thus reducing the impacts of stress, including oats, sweet potatoes, walnuts, maple syrup, pastured chicken, seaweed, and dark leafy greens, among others. Fermented foods such as sauerkraut, kimchi, miso, and unsweetened yogurt are especially supportive in mitigating the effects of chronic stress because they feed beneficial gut bacteria that secrete the hormones we need to support a healthy stress response. Find the whole foods that feel both wholesome and comforting to you. These are your personal stress reducers.

Breathwork

One of the best ways to destress is to breathe. I like to use mealtimes as an opportunity to practice deep breathing. Not only does this practice help the body digest better, but it also takes the nervous system out of chronic stress mode.

Some simple breathing exercises I have found helpful include the following.

~ Balanced Breathing

This practice balances the two hemispheres of the brain. If counting doesn't resonate for you, try taking three deep breaths that start and end in the belly.

1. Sit down. Take a deep breath in and out.
2. Breathe in for four counts.
3. Hold the breath for two counts.
4. Breathe out for four counts.
5. Hold the breath for two counts.
6. Repeat this cycle three times.

~ 4-7-8 Breath

A breathwork practice that helps me relax was popularized by Dr. Andrew Weil, founder and director of the Center for Integrative Medicine at the University of Arizona. It is called the 4-7-8 breath and its relaxing effects are due to the exhale lasting longer than the inhale.

1. Sit down. Bring your awareness to your breath.
2. Exhale through your mouth, pulling your navel in toward your spine to release as much air as possible.
3. Close your mouth and inhale through your nose for four counts.
4. Hold the breath for seven counts.
5. Exhale through your mouth for eight counts.
6. Repeat this cycle three times.

Breathwork to Address Cravings

Many of us eat for reasons other than hunger. Perhaps when we are hit by stress or we are feeling lonely, we might reach for something tasty to trigger the reward and pleasure centers of the brain. But is it food that we truly seek? Eating can be comforting when we have been challenged emotionally. Sometimes emotional eating is exactly what's needed, even though its support is transient. At other times, other forms of emotional support, like connection with other people or with nature, can offer longer-lasting benefits.

Many of us know what our triggers are. Triggers are useful information on the path to healing because they remind us of how challenging it can be to live in a body in the world in this lifetime. When trying to heal, whether physically and emotionally, it is important to know that we can respond to triggers in various ways. How does it feel to take a deep breath when you're feeling triggered? Food triggers—those situations, thoughts, or feelings that initiate a food craving—usually last less than a minute. What would it be like to take a deep breath before reaching for comfort food? The more we breathe deeply, the more our nervous system relaxes. The more it relaxes, the less we feel the need to satisfy a fleeting craving.

Before reaching for comfort food, try one of the simple breathing techniques discussed here. You might then find that you are not actually hungry. Or, if you still feel hungry, you might make choices that continue to amplify the feeling of calm presence that can arise after deep breathing.

~ The Wim Hof Method

Dutch extreme athlete Wim Hof developed a signature technique that combines the hermetic stress of exposure to cold water with breathwork practices. Scientists researching Hof's method have found that these two strategies together strengthen immunity, improve sleep and energy, and balance anxiety and depression. Wim Hof encourages folks to start with the following:

1. For the last 15 seconds or so of a shower, adjust the water temperature to full cold.
2. Stand under the water while taking three to five deep breaths.

If you would like to try more breathwork practices, many resources are available. See James Nestor's book *Breath,* which offers a deep dive into the science and practice of breathwork. There also are many incredible breathwork teachers out there, including Jasmine Marie, Dr. Angel Acosta, Chauna Bryant, Jennifer Patterson, and more.

INTUITIVE EATING

In 1995, nutrition therapists Elyse Resch and Evelyn Tribole wrote one of the first books on the concept of intuitive eating. That book sparked a worldwide awareness that the mentality of dieting disrupts metabolic health and leads to stress and disordered eating. Tribole herself went from being a dietician who endorsed diet culture to finding her path as a guide for patients in finding their own ideal way to eat. Intuitive eating reminds us to be compassionate with ourselves and each other, to approach eating with nonjudgment, to honor hunger and fullness, to respect genetics and body type, and to reject diet culture.

The word *diet* comes from the Greek *diaita,* meaning "a way of life." It's time to reappropriate this word and use it as it was originally intended, not as the restrictive and dysregulating framework it has become. As Resch explains, "It's time to let go of a dieting system that is toxic. The data show that 95% of people who go on diets fail at them. . . . The only alternative is to start trusting the body and feeling the freedom and enjoyment of food that comes with that."[1] Our capacity to enjoy food has been smothered by the fast-paced nature of modern life. When we start to slow down and truly savor our meals, we can tap into the body's intuition about the foods that are ideal at any given time.

The wide availability of industrially processed food choices in the United States is not our fault. We are subject to the whims of CEOs who want to make more profit for their companies and the pharmaceutical industry at the expense of public health. Where I grew up in Italy, folks who did not have high earnings gained their nourishment and abundance from growing their own food. *Cucina povera* is now widely popular in Italy because this peasant food, made with whole, simple ingredients, is often the most delicious. In an article about the current epidemic of diet-related diseases, cardiologist Dariush Mozaffarian concludes, "Industrialization of our food appears to be a core contributor to harmful biological adaptations."[2]

I have seen my young children be very clear about when they are full or choose to eat certain parts of a meal and not others, like skipping the rice on their plate even though the previous day they had eaten all of it. I believe that this instinct arises in part from their whole foods diet, which allows their microbiomes to remain intact and send clear messages to their brains about nourishment. In addition, they trust their intuition and follow their needs for nourishment in each moment. Many of us were raised to be part of something like the "clean plate club." This kind of framework takes people away from their hunger and satiety cues and creates a sense of guilt or accomplishment around clearing a plate. Instead, intuitive eating encourages people to tune in to the nutritional value of food, the pleasure it brings to the senses, and feelings of fullness, which can change at different times. Just as with mindful eating, this way of relating intuitively to food supports both mental and digestive health.

I still hear the voice of my dad saying things like, "Don't eat too much bread or it will make you fat." Whether he was conscious of it or not, my dad was repeating admonitions he had likely heard from his mother. My dad and his mother were wonderful guides for eating well; they gave me the crucial foundation in food as medicine and folk herbalism that inspires me to this day. But they, too, had been indoctrinated with some of the dietary strictures of the world around them, and the messages they sometimes passed along created associations in my subconscious mind, like "bread equals fat." I now know intellectually that is not true. However, I needed to reprogram myself to appreciate the potent nourishment of a whole-grain bread made with love and appreciation of ancestry. As an homage to such bread, I wrote a poem in the ghazal style, which originated in Arabic poetry centuries ago.

Bread Ghazal

My father taught me that fenugreek, caraway,
and fennel are the secrets to our rye bread.
Hard enough to crack under a fist,
this bread is called by its German name: schuettelbrot.
Every fall, we stocked Nonna's cellar
with newspaper-wrapped stacks of this hardtack bread.
After moving to the States, I spent a year researching
the Roma, who carried spices in their caravans for
    bread.
They brought fenugreek, caraway, and fennel
from north Asia, wouldn't let those seeds drop
until they reached a safe place to bake their moro.
The Alps became this haven, and rye sourdough
has been handed down ever since, bubbling
into the staple with which we were bred.
When I go home to Italy, grains are not the villains
they have become for America's
health-obsessed disdainers of bread.

Instead, they are revered as keepers
at the chapel door of seasons: there is strength
to persevere if one at least has bread.

In her book *The Body Is Not an Apology,* Sonya Renee Taylor exposes the truth about the current oppressive society that disconnects us from our true selves. When we reconnect to self-love, she says, "we feel inspired to awaken others and to interrupt the systems that perpetuate body shame and oppression against all bodies. When we act from this truth on a global scale, we usher in the transformative opportunity of radical self-love, which is the opportunity for a more just, equitable, and compassionate world for us all." Instead of listening to what's being preached by others, we can choose to look within and ask ourselves where our beliefs about ourselves came from and whether they need to be updated.

The body is truly not something for which to apologize; it is our greatest gift and our best tool for liberation. I know from personal and professional experience that it is possible to shift what we eat to promote our unique version of wellness by heeding the body's messages for nourishment. When health is the goal and present moment awareness is the mindset, transformation can truly take place.

The word *intuition* comes from the Latin *in* and *tueri,* meaning "to look within." *Intellect,* from the Latin *inter* and *legere,* means "to choose between." The mind uses discernment, and the soul knows the inner truth. By weaving intuition and intellect, we perform the radical act of restoring the connection between humans and Earth. *Radical,* after all, comes from the Latin *radix,* "root." It is time to root in the ever-changing, profound wisdom of self-knowledge informed by nature. In *The Art of the Commonplace* Wendell Berry says, "Only by restoring the broken connections can we be healed. Connection is health. And what our society does its best to disguise from us is how ordinary, how commonly attainable, health is. We lose our health—and create profitable diseases and dependencies—by failing to see the direct connections between living and eating, eating and working, working and loving."

THE NEED FOR RITUAL

When working toward finding true wellness, traditional healing modalities that are still practiced today encourage folks to include not only the body and mind but also the spirit in the practice of healing. As the pace of life increases, rituals support us in slowing down. When we light a candle and offer thanks before a meal, the process of eating takes on a different feeling and pace. Ideally, we feel more connected to the present moment and what's happening right now. As a child in Catholic school, I frequently attended Mass with the nuns before going home to eat lunch. My classmates and I would take turns swinging the frankincense censer and lighting candles before reciting prayers.

Even though I no longer practice religious rituals, I bring the spirit of what was offered to me growing up into my life. These kinds of spiritual practices bring us into a sense of flow, into a space where there is no thinking, just immersion in the experience at hand. The word *ritual* comes from the Latin *rituo,* meaning "to do again." The repetitive nature of rituals allows the mind, body, and spirit to align in this flow and feel the freedom that comes from structure. The most supportive habits ultimately become rituals.

Rituals allow us to truly enjoy all of life's gifts. They bring the power of awareness, which creates an opportunity for choice. If I am moving mindlessly through my day, just "going through the motions," I limit my choices and thus limit my growth. When a ritual slows me down, I start to notice that I have been operating under preestablished patterns. Now I can choose either to continue living inside those patterns or to change them. Awareness precedes change. If you want to change the flow of your day, the way you eat, the way you move, or the way you relate to yourself and others, bring in a ritual to catalyze that change. The ritual creates space; the space lets change unfold.

An adage to which I often turn is "work is paying attention to what matters most." Rituals help us focus our attention on the parts of life that feel meaningful so that we can enhance the experience of being human.

Creating a ritual is much like creating a habit. It's easiest to start small by adding a ritual to something you already do, like eating. Giving thanks for food before eating it, for example, can provide the opportunity to create a habit that becomes a ritual. This kind of gratitude ritual can support us in making shifts in our eating habits.

Consumer culture teaches judgment. Whether positive or negative, judgment is judgment. When judgment is used to discern what's needed in a particular situation, it can be helpful. However, the mind has millions of thoughts and makes millions of judgments daily. Many of these judgments are self-criticisms. Can you hear your internal voice? What does it sound like? Mine often sounds like "you ate too much chocolate" or "why didn't you finish that project today?" or "don't you need to get more exercise?" Although these voices are trying to help me achieve my potential, they are not kind. The more negative self-talk I hear, the more I feel deflated and like I lack the capacity to be who I want to be.

A gratitude practice transforms the way we think about and see ourselves. Whether it's offering thanks for the food we are eating or listing three things for which we are grateful before bed, expressing gratitude helps our conscious and unconscious mind move from negative judgment and criticism to focusing on the things that we appreciate about life. Because much of modern society has a negativity bias and news messages are often fear-based, trying to shift to a nonjudgmental mindset can feel like we are going against the grain. Many of us were raised by caregivers who openly criticized and worried about most aspects of life; this kind of modeled behavior can be externalized, seen for what it is, and released.

Part of this release involves processing grief and past trauma. Many spiritual traditions believe that, to practice gratitude, we must first explore our grief, and there are a number of beautiful ways to do so. The Dagara tradition of West Africa, for example, offers powerful grieving rituals. Sobonfu Somé, a Burkinabe author and teacher of ancestral wisdom and indigenous spiritual practices who is rooted in the Dagara tribal tradition, wrote about loss, wisdom, and family relationships. Martín Prechtel teaches from the Maya indigenous perspective about grief and praise. He tells the story of going to the ocean when filled with grief and offering his grief to the ocean all night long, until the sunrise brought him to tears, and he began to sing songs of gratitude to the ocean for its healing powers. Some Mexican cultures believe that La Virgen de Guadalupe, the Mother of Sorrows, can take all grief into her cloak of stars and transform it. Dagara, Maya, and Catholic traditions all believe in offering food as a way to honor grief and allow it be transformed. There are many more indigenous and religious grief and praise practices. I am naming just a few that I know.

When I studied Diné traditions at Diné College, on Diné land in Arizona, one of the rituals we learned to practice was the corn offering. We would wake up at dawn and walk sunwise to offer corn flour in each of the directions while singing the song of the sacred mountains, which hold each direction and offer a safe container in which the Diné can thrive. This practice reflects a reverence for nature as well as the awareness that everything is alive, changing, and deserving of praise. It also reminds us that with change comes loss, and the offering allows for grieving all that has been lost.

We must grieve the loss of people, places, experiences, foods, and memories to rekindle praise and gratitude for life. The water of our tears puts out the fire of grief and offers a path forward. Grief is a natural response to loss or change of any kind. It is neither a pathological condition nor a personality disorder. Conflicting feelings caused by changes in something familiar can lead to grief. Even a positive change can require grief. Weaning a baby from breast milk is an example that comes to mind for me. As much as my babies and I were ready to move on from this daily ritual that was nourishing for everyone, there was a time to let go. By grieving the loss through a weaning ceremony, I was able to find peace in witnessing the inevitable growth of my children. Reflect on ways that you can put your grief to rest so that you can be well. Grief is energy. Energy can be moved and transformed.

Here is a ritual that I learned while studying a program called Unbodying White Bodied Supremacy with the SUSU CommUNITY Farm in Vermont.[3] I have used this grief ritual with myself and my family: Write down what you are grieving on paper. Put those pieces of paper in a beautiful box. Cry, pray, and sit with the box. Give it offerings of candles, food, herbs, ash, water, salt, or other things from nature. Give thanks to the box, and then burn it or offer it to the earth. Now you have cleared a space inside yourself for gratitude to arise.

SHIFTING HABITS

When we make a shift toward a mindset of gratitude, we become like a plant turning toward the light. We reach for the things that fill our hearts with joy and thereby bring more gratitude into our lives. It may sound simple, but switching our mindset is key to shifting our habits. When we do not love and appreciate ourselves, we are more likely to continue perpetuating unhelpful habits because we are self-sabotaging.

Simpatias are behavior-change rituals that have roots in the Brazilian Macumba spiritual tradition. From galvanizing an abundance mentality to helping people quit smoking, *simpatias* create a framework for behavior change that feels supportive and meaningful. A wide-reaching study on *simpatias* found that the more intricate and repetitive the rituals are, the more effective they seem to be in helping people change a behavior.[4]

As we have seen, rituals can be helpful in supporting a behavior change or new habit. The more we incorporate practices like mindfulness and intuitive eating into daily life, the more they become a ritual that creates space to move beyond the rational. Habits can then become gateways into our intuition, reminders to move from the guidance of the truth within. Rituals may look different from person to person, perhaps stemming from childhood experiences or from practices rooted in our heritage that feel in alignment.

Acknowledge Mistakes as Signs of Progress

Shifting a habit is not always easy. Science says that it takes twenty-one days on average to develop a new habit. We do not strive for perfection; we aim for progress. But if we slip into an old pattern, it doesn't mean that we need to throw all our efforts out the window and return to negative thinking or self-judgment. Instead, it means that we are human. We are living a life of perfect imperfection. We are honoring that our mistakes indicate our progress.

When I make a mistake, I see it as an affirmation that I am working on making a change. I am in a process. Mistakes are signposts along the path of transformation. They are reminding me to slow down, take stock, figure out why I slipped up.

As an example, I set a goal to stop eating chocolate for thirty days. But then, somewhere in the middle of that time, I ate chocolate. I ate that chocolate because my daughter had a fever, my partner's car broke down, my infant threw food all over the dining room wall, and I forgot to call my friend on his birthday. I ate that chocolate because I was stressed. When I look at my day and understand my stress, I can have compassion for myself. I can remind myself that tomorrow is another day. Not all is lost because I did not meet my goal on one day. When I did eat chocolate, I was mindful of why I was putting it in my body. I appreciated the flavor, texture, richness, and soothing quality of this food. And I realized that I needed to incorporate into my life more stress reduction tools that didn't involve eating chocolate.

Starting a Habit-Shifting Practice

Pick one habit that you would like to shift during the next three months. It could be food related or not. Here are some ideas:

- Shift from eating a snack as a work break to taking a ten-minute walk as a work break.
- Shift from eating in front of a computer to eating at a table and taking a deep breath before meals.
- Shift from jumping out of bed and rushing out the door to waking up fifteen minutes earlier and getting grounded for the day.
- Shift from being on a screen before bedtime to listing three things for which you are grateful before bedtime.
- Shift from eating processed foods to veggies and nuts as snacks.

- Shift from using refined cane sugar to using maple syrup as a sweetener.

To begin, redirect the habit you want to shift. With the example of my habit of eating chocolate, I can first appreciate that it's not the worst thing in the world. However, I am eating chocolate when I am tired and stressed. The issue isn't the chocolate. It's the need for rest and nurturing. Try to identify the core issue related to your habit. Do you need support for your adrenals? Do you need more rest, movement, or breathwork? Do you need to balance your blood glucose levels?

Once you have identified the root cause of the habit you would like to shift, find something to take its place. Now, when I crave chocolate, I sit down and take a deep breath. I try to make my exhale longer than my inhale. Then I do something totally unrelated to food. I put on a specific song and dance to it. My kids love joining in the fun! Thanks to my desire to shift this habit, we have created a family ritual of picking a song and having a dance party after dinner. This satisfies my need to release stress and enjoy life with my family and has replaced the perceived need for chocolate. In addition, I go to bed thirty minutes earlier on days when I am feeling stressed. This is true nourishment.

How do you want to redirect your habit? Choose something that you can do quickly and easily that doesn't relate to the habit you would like to shift. For example, try putting on a song and dancing, going into a different room and picking up an art project or a musical instrument, laying down on the floor and stretching, or burning a candle or diffusing an essential oil.

Start noticing how many times a day you gravitate toward your habit and how many times you choose to redirect instead. I keep a piece of paper on my desk with two columns: one for how many times I felt my habit come up (eat chocolate) and one for how many times I redirected (dance). It's great to look at that page and see where progress is happening. What we focus on expands. Taking note helps us expand our capacity to shift a habit.

Behavioral psychologist B. J. Fogg's book *Tiny Habits* is based on human behavior research that has led him to create tools for shaping long-term change where, as he writes, we can "have an epiphany, change our environment, or change our habits in tiny ways [take baby steps]." (Visit the Tiny Habits website to explore resources.) The more we take charge of how we want to relate to our food, our days, and our world, the more we become empowered to heal ourselves through the daily activities that shape our lives. The more we choose to make the mundane feel sacred, the more meaning we source from simple acts like walking up the stairs or tying shoes. When we are present with whatever is happening in the moment, we can transform stress into joy.

5

Trusting Your Gut

How Microbiomes Interact

The human body is an elaborate vessel optimized for the growth and spread of our microbial inhabitants.

JUSTIN SONNENBURG

After I left the outside world and went underground to embark on my healing journey, parasites began to prey on my nervous and endocrine systems. Joy was replaced by stress. Different practitioners had recommendations for me that were confusing or conflicting. I felt paralyzed by all the noise. I developed a disordered eating pattern known as orthorexia, from the Greek words meaning "fear of food." I reduced my safe foods to brown rice, homemade sourdough rye bread, kale, chicken, olive oil, and salt. I quickly realized that this fear-based approach was not life-affirming. It felt more comfortable to stick with what was familiar, yet I knew that the only constant in life is change. Although my intellect understood that I needed to do things differently, my intuition still resided in a traumatized space.

To support the process of looking at my trauma, I called upon my grandmother, Aldina Masé. She passed in Italy on the same April day that I contracted parasites in Bali. I recollected her teachings about wildcrafting, herbal medicine-making, and food preservation. Her wisdom served as a balm for my fear and a pathway toward trusting my intuition again. Slowly, I returned to the culinary and herbal practices with which I was raised. This poem reminds me of all that she taught my cousins, my brother, and me when we were growing up.

Origins

Brother, you slide an Amarone bottled in 1992
from your Vermont farmhouse wine rack,
where it dutifully collects telling dust.
It's ten years old and could age another ten.
"Dalla cantina di Nonna Dina": You name our
*   grandmother's cellar,*
cool even in summer's noon.
I remember being sent down there to fetch something,
how dread and delight seized me as I imagined
what might lurk behind that oak door:
mold-mottled sausages dangling from top shelves
from which Fontina wheels with butter-dulled rinds
*   would peer;*
shiny jars of apricot jam, proud brown bottles of
*   elderberry syrup,*
dried wild mushrooms bagged in muslin, and crusty
*   rye bread wrapped in newspaper—*
all preserved with the patience of mountains.
There, gleaming with egg wash on the marble worktable,
I would spot my charge: crostata di mele.
Bravely I carried the apple tart upstairs.
When you show me this wine in your kitchen,
I remember the flavor of apples picked that morning,
the melt of spring butter over latticed crust,
and a grandmother who splashed wine into our water
to make us stronger.

As I returned to the wisdom imparted by Nonna Dina, I grated vegetables from our garden, sprinkled them with salt, pounded them in a bowl, and filled jars to ferment for probiotic benefit. I walked through the meadows behind our home and wild-crafted perennial plants like red clover to flush the lymph, St. John's wort to support mental health, yarrow to heal the gut lining and reduce stomach cramps, and Japanese knotweed to eradicate gut pathogens. I started growing *Artemisia annua,* which is indigenous to China and is called *qing hao* in Chinese. Travelers must have brought the fragrant branches with them to use as an antiparasitic, because this plant also grows wild in Europe today.

I began to heal myself by striking a balance between eradicating parasites and supporting gut health. Where antibiotics sterilize, this approach heals the root causes of disease. I also started learning about healing modalities from other parts of the world, and that is how I began to explore the significance of enteric types in the healing process.

ENTEROTYPING

It's no wonder that we have an expression about "trusting your gut." Our intestines act as a kind of primordial brain that governs many of our body's processes. Beyond physiological wellness, what we eat and how we eat it affects our immunity and mood. Food choices matter. Gut bacteria can change in a few days depending on whether we eat more protein, fat, or carbohydrates. Science has endeavored to understand the human gut microbiome in relationship to its external environment just as traditional healing systems explore the relationship between constitution and conditions. This scientific exploration is known as metagenomics, the study of genetic material sampled directly from the environment. This study includes the internal environment of human beings, which can be classified by enterotype.[1]

Meta = beyond
Genome = the genetic material of an organism
Entero = relating to the intestines

Researchers in an international consortium, including Jeroen Raes of the Flanders Institute in Belgium, assessed human stool samples to classify people into three primary enterotypes, or bacterial ecosystems: *Bacteroides, Prevotella,* and *Ruminococcus.*[2]

We are all ecosystems. Just as the underground mycorrhizal network of mushroom mycelia creates large webs of connection, the human gut microbiome allows different parts of the body to communicate with one another. Of all the DNA we carry around, only a small percentage of it is human. The other DNA belongs to the billions of microbes that live in our gut, among other places. Many are bacteria that take advantage of the protection and food we offer them while making vitamins and digestive enzymes that are essential to the smooth functioning of our body and mind. Each of these three enterotype bacterial ecosystems does things slightly differently. The *Bacteroides* ecosystem consists largely of bacteria that get energy by fermenting sugars and proteins. The *Prevotella* ecosystem contains a lot of microbes that digest proteins in the mucus lining of the gut. *Ruminococcus,* the most common type, prefer both gut mucus proteins and simple sugars.

In addition to their different food preferences, these enterotype groups also have different output profiles. The *Bacteroides* type makes vitamins, while *Prevotella* is good at making folic acid and thiamin. Although scientists are not yet sure whether enterotypes result from the place we live or the food we eat, research is starting to reveal that common traits, such as body mass index, can be markers for enterotypes. Different enterotypes also respond to stress and to seasonal changes in different ways.[3]

It can be helpful to know more about your enterotype because it affects which foods are ideal for you. If you would like, you can conduct testing through companies such as the Nutrition Genome. Alternatively, by noticing what you eat and how you digest it, you are more likely to be able to identify your enterotype. Keep a food journal that also includes information about the consistency, frequency, and type of your stool. Try it for a week and see what you discover. To learn more about global microbiome diversity and look at microbial maps that represent microbial connections worldwide, you can visit the Earth Microbiome Project website. As stated on their website, they have collected extensive data "to understand patterns in microbial ecology across the biomes and habitats of our planet."

The Enteric Nervous System

The body's enteric nervous system (ENS) contains more than 500 million neurons and is embedded in the lining of the digestive tract from the esophagus to the anus. It has been described as a second brain because it operates autonomously and uses many neurotransmitters that secrete most of the body's stress and relaxation hormones. It communicates with the central nervous system (CNS) via the vagus nerve. The ENS's neurons allows it to transport reflexes and support the body if the CNS is not responsive. These neurons control peristalsis, the muscular contractions that churn food and move it through the intestines.

The enteric nervous system changes its function based on the nutrients found in the food we eat. The study of the interface between nutrition and genetic composition is referred to as nutrigenomics. This branch of biology explores how the food we eat can alter our gut microbiome as well as turn genes on and off. Michael Fenech, a research scientist at the CSIRO Genome Health and Nutrigenomics Laboratory in Adelaide, Australia, explains that "the main goal of [nutrigenomics] is to define the optimal dietary intake . . . to maintain damage to the genome at its lowest possible level."[4] In other words, food is truly a health intervention because it can instruct the body to either enter a disease process or prevent it. Eating our own unique set of ideal foods is not only essential for a healthy gut but also has a huge impact on maintaining whole body health.

How Gut Bacteria Affect Mood

The ideal balance of gut flora can have a positive influence on mental health. The study that jump-started researchers' deeper inquiries into the connection between gut flora and mood took place at Kyushu University in Japan in 2004. The researchers showed that sterile mice—those that had never encountered microbes—produced twice the amount of stress hormones as other mice when exposed to a stressful situation. Scientists deduced that gut bacteria influenced the release of stress hormones.[5] We now know that neurotransmitters that line the intestines are responsible for producing a great deal of our stress hormones, including both the "fight or flight" sympathetic hormones and the "rest and digest" parasympathetic hormones.

The gut microbiome and the brain communicate through a system called the microbiota-gut-brain axis, which itself relies heavily on the vagus nerve, the longest nerve in the autonomic nervous system.[6] Positive emotions build vagus nerve strength, and a strong vagus nerve helps generate positive emotions.[7] Keeping the vagus nerve toned is crucial to maintaining balanced mood and cognitive health. We can support vagal tone both by supporting the gut with prebiotic and probiotic foods and by reducing stress through practices like breathwork, movement, and mindfulness. Because the vagus nerve modulates the gut-brain axis, it is important to help the nervous system transition into parasympathetic mode, or "rest and digest" mode, to strengthen the vagus nerve. Simple exercises like turning the head to look first to the left, then to the right, then up, and then down support the nervous system in feeling like it is safe to relax and be present.

Certain foods also support nervous system regulation by soothing or rebuilding frayed myelin sheathing at the ends of nerves. I crafted the following recipe when feeling particularly anxious. After researching ingredients like chicken broth, coconut, and sweet potato, I learned why I was intuitively reaching for those foods: they help heal nerve endings.

🍎 Chicken and Sweet Potato Stew

    2 tablespoons coconut oil
    I small red or yellow onion, finely chopped
    4 cloves garlic, minced
    I pound chicken tenders (hormone and antibiotic-free)
    I medium sweet potato, chopped
    I tablespoon chopped fresh ginger

½ teaspoon ground cinnamon

½ teaspoon ground turmeric

½ teaspoon sea salt

1 cup full-fat canned coconut milk

3 cups chicken broth

5 ounces baby spinach

1 tablespoon fresh lemon or lime juice

Heat the oil in a stock pot. Add the onion and garlic and sauté on medium low heat, stirring occasionally, until the onion has softened, about 5 minutes.

Scootch the onion off to the side of the pot and add the chicken. Allow the chicken to brown for 2 to 3 minutes, then flip it over and let it brown on the other side for 1 to 2 minutes.

Add the chopped sweet potato, fresh ginger, cinnamon, turmeric, and sea salt. Stir well.

Pour in the coconut milk and chicken broth and add the baby spinach. Cover the pot, bring the soup to a full boil, then reduce the heat to low and simmer for 15 minutes, or until the sweet potato is cooked through.

Stir in the lemon or lime juice. Let cook, uncovered, for 5 to 10 minutes. Taste the soup for flavor and add more salt and lemon or lime juice, if needed.

THE MICROBIOME AND WELLNESS

As infants, our guts colonize with beneficial bacteria, which secrete bioactive compounds that affect our physiology and metabolism. These bacteria have a symbiotic relationship with the human body and are crucial to maintaining homeostasis, or balance, in our systems. A healthy microbiome leads to strong immunity, balanced blood sugar, regulated cholesterol, and good mental health, among other things. Medication, stress, food choices, and disease can negatively affect the natural colonies of gut bacteria. Certain foods, on the other hand, can maintain or repopulate our beneficial gut microflora.

Prebiotics are those foods we eat that, in turn, feed our gut microflora. They mainly comprise the dietary fiber found in legumes, fruits, vegetables, and whole grains. Some good sources of prebiotics are apples, artichokes, asparagus, avocado, flaxseed, banana, dandelion greens, leeks, oats, and unsweetened cacao. One of my favorite prebiotic food sources is apple cider vinegar. It helps balance blood glucose as well as being wonderful for enhancing pancreatic enzyme secretions and nourishing gut flora. (Note: avoid apple cider vinegar if you have yeast overgrowth, but otherwise, enjoy it.)

Postbiotics are the metabolites of gut microflora, or the components that result from intestinal microbes consuming prebiotic fiber. Though they are wastes of a sort, postbiotics directly lead to many health benefits for the body, such as reducing inflammation, preventing irritable bowel syndrome (IBS), and maintaining balanced blood glucose. If you want to get more postbiotics, eat more probiotic foods.

Probiotics are those foods that themselves contain the very same microbes we need for a healthy microbiome. Eating probiotics repopulates our gut microflora. They help strengthen the body's barrier against infection, as well as boosting the antibacterial, immune-modulating, and anti-inflammatory aspects of a healthy gut. You can gain probiotic benefit from foods like yogurt, kefir, kombucha, tempeh, miso, sauerkraut, and kimchi. Do you know which ones are indigenous to your ancestral food traditions? I grew up with sauerkraut as well as jars of *giardiniera,* lacto-fermented onions, peppers, celery, carrots, and cauliflower. Just as with pickles, giardiniera, whose name means "gardener," can be either lacto-fermented with salt and time or quickly pickled with vinegar. The quick-pickled version of this gut-balancing condiment is known in Italy as *sottaceto,* "under vinegar."

It seems like everyone is recommending probiotic supplements these days. In 2001, a ground-breaking research study was published in *Science* magazine explaining that we can augment the beneficial bacteria in our body by taking broad-strain probiotic supplements. As important as this discovery was, it did not consider what we now know: Just as we have a blood type, we have an enteric type. Some probiotic strains might not be good for certain enteric types. Sometimes, broad-spectrum probiotic supplements can do more harm than good because they're trying to grow colonies of bacteria that a particular gut doesn't support. For this reason, I recommend getting probiotic support from food. With food, the body is better able to take what it needs and leave the rest behind.

There are some situations in which a therapeutic probiotic strain might be indicated. For example, after a course of antibiotics, I recommend taking a high-quality probiotic like Ther-Biotic Complete from Klaire Labs. For someone experiencing gut permeability, also known as leaky gut syndrome, supplements containing *Akkermansia muciniphila* and *Lacticaseibacillus rhamnosus* can help restore the gut lining. *Limosilactobacillus reuteri* supports the body's innate capacity to grow its own healthy colonies of beneficial gut flora and thus promotes a healthy immune response;[8] it lives in the small intestine as well as the large intestine, which means that it also supports sleep and oxytocin production. These strains are resistant to bile acids in the stomach, which means that they can safely travel to the small intestine to offer healing support to the gut lining. A strain called *Saccharomyces boulardii* is effective in eradicating *Helicobacter pylori* bacteria, which can lead to dysbiosis and SIBO (small intestinal bacterial overgrowth). *S. boulardii* is antibiotic resistant, thus a good strain to use for those who need to take antibiotics.

The strain *Aspergillus oryzae* can help degrade excess mold in the system caused by ochratoxin, which is present primarily in grains, legumes, and coffee beans that have not been stored properly. *Lactobacillus helveticus* boosts mood and helps the nervous system adapt to stress. *L. rhamnosus* is a profound blood sugar balancer and helps reduce the body's tendency toward insulin resistance. It can be supportive to type 2 diabetics and Parkinson's disease patients. *Lactiplantibacillus plantarum* is abundant in lacto-fermented vegetables like sauerkraut and kimchi. It lines the intestinal wall and keeps pathogens and undigested food from leaking into the bloodstream.

Streptococcus salivarius is excellent for preventing upper respiratory infections and can be supportive during cold and flu season. It colonizes everyone's mouth, regardless of enteric type. *Bifidobacterium longum* supports healthy fat metabolism and has been shown to help balance cholesterol. *Bifidobacterium bifidum* and *Lacticaseibacillus paracasei* are excellent for liver and skin health. *Bifidobacterium lactis* is helpful for weight management and blood glucose balance.[9]

These are just a few examples to help elucidate how intelligent and specialized nature is, both within the body and in its surroundings. In a world where probiotic supplements tend to prevail, it's important to remember that, just like antibiotics, these are concentrated strains have specific applications. It's ideal to get probiotic benefit from food and use specific strains therapeutically with the support of a practitioner.

Probiotic foods are highly concentrated; a spoonful or forkful goes a long way. If you notice gas or bloating from eating fermented foods, eat less of them or use them less frequently until your body acclimates to them. Try having a spoonful of miso stirred into a cup of hot water. Miso is fermented soybean paste, a traditional food from Asia that is still fermented today in large containers that are sometimes buried underground. Drinking a cup of miso can be a great way to beat an afternoon craving for sweets or refined flour products like baked goods.

LACTO-FERMENTATION: CREATING OUR OWN CULTURE

For centuries, humans worldwide used lactic acid fermentation to preserve their vegetables. Since the advent of industrial food production, these foods have nearly disappeared. It is important to revive this traditional knowledge and reap its benefits, which include the following:

- **Active cultures and enzymes.** As with those found in yogurt, the probiotics and enzymes in traditional lacto-fermented foods are known to support proper digestion, aid in nutrient absorption, contribute to healthy metabolic function, and inhibit harmful microbes in the intestinal system.

- **Lactic acid.** This primary by-product of fermentation supports the growth of essential intestinal flora, normalizes acid levels in the stomach, helps the body assimilate proteins and iron, and stimulates cell metabolism.

- **Improved nutrient availability.** Natural fermentation breaks down phytic acid in food, which blocks mineral absorption. One study found significantly better absorption of iron by humans from a mix of lacto-fermented vegetables as compared to the same mix of fresh vegetables.

- **Cultural creativity.** As fermentation master Sandor Katz explains, when working with the bacterial cultures that occur naturally in the air to make a lacto-fermented food, an inter-relationship develops between the internal human ecosystem and that of the surrounding air. Thus, a "culture" is developed that, when consumed, makes humans even more local to where they live.

Soaking Grains and Legumes

You can ferment any grain or legume by soaking it for up to twenty-four hours in a pot with water and ¼ teaspoon salt per cup of soaking water. This traditional practice allows for the fermentation process to predigest certain fibers. After soaking, drain as best as you can. Some water can remain in the pot. Refill the pot with fresh water and cook your grain or legume. While this practice doesn't maintain the probiotics of the fermentation process (because the grain and legumes are then cooked), it does increases nutrient availability, reduce the content of gas-producing phytic acid, and cut down on cooking time.

Kimchi

Every summer, my family makes our version of kimchi, a traditional Korean ferment of vegetables. We set up an outdoor table with cutting boards, knives, bowls, and graters and then get to work processing vegetables. Everyone picks a station to start with, and we switch when we feel like it. We harvest carrots, daikon, Napa cabbage, leeks, chiles, and radishes from our garden to include in the mix.

Kimchi is much like the Italian giardiniera; the main difference is that giardiniera tends to use bell peppers instead of cabbage or bok choy. Feel free to incorporate other veggies into this kimchi, if you like, such as beans or peas, cauliflower, eggplant, Jerusalem artichokes, okra, squash, or turnips.

1 pound Napa cabbage, Savoy cabbage, and/or bok choy, coarsely chopped

1 daikon radish or a few red radishes, sliced into crescents

2 carrots, sliced into crescents

1 onion or leek (and/or a few shallots or scallions), chopped

1 head garlic, cloves separated, peeled, and chopped

3 or 4 chiles (or to taste), chopped

6-inch piece of dulse or other seaweed, cut with scissors

3 tablespoon (or more) grated fresh ginger

1 tablespoon salt

Combine the cabbage, radish, carrots, onion, garlic, chiles, seaweed, ginger, and salt in a large bowl. Mix well.

Stuff the mixture into a wide-mouth quart jar. Pack it in tightly, adding more of the veggie mixture and pressing down until the juices squeeze out of the veggies. With the salt, these juices make a brine. The veggies must be submerged in liquid to prevent mold from growing.

Cover the jar with a napkin or a piece of cheesecloth secured with a rubber band.

Put the jar in a big bowl to catch any liquids that might bubble up from spilling onto the counter.

Let the kimchi sit at room temperature (60° to 70°F is preferred) for I week to 10 days, until it reaches your desired flavor and texture. The longer the vegetables ferment, the more sour they will become.

Allow the mixture to sit for about a week in a warm place. Press the kimchi down each day so the veggies at the top get submerged in the brine.

The longer the kimchi ferments, the more sour it will become.

When it tastes sour and pungent enough for you, store it in the fridge.

🍎 Lacto-Fermented Carrots

4 cups coarsely grated carrots

I tablespoon grated fresh ginger

I tablespoon salt

In a medium bowl, mix the carrots, ginger, and sea salt. Knead with clean hands until the carrots have released enough liquid to cover themselves.

Transfer the mixture to a wide-mouth glass quart jar, pressing the mixture down to submerge it completely underneath the liquid.

Put the jar in a big bowl to catch any liquids that might bubble up from spilling onto the counter.

Cover the jar with a napkin or a piece of cheesecloth secured with a rubber band.

Let the carrots sit at room temperature (60° to 70°F is preferred) for I week to 10 days, until they reach your desired flavor and texture. The longer they ferment, the more sour they will become.

Check the carrots daily, as you would check on a plant or a pet. Using a fork, press the carrots below the surface of the liquid brine to prevent any mold from developing.

Once the carrots are finished, put a tight lid on the jar and move to the refrigerator. The flavor will continue to develop as they age in the fridge.

Tempeh

Tempeh is a highly digestible relative of tofu. It's made from soybeans that are fermented with beneficial *Rhizopus* mold. It is difficult to absorb most of the protein from soy foods unless they are fermented. Indigenous to Indonesia, tempeh is more flavorful than tofu and provides incredible nutritional benefit. I will never forget stepping into the cool, volcanic tempeh fermentation caves in Gianyar, Bali. The tropical heat outside is erased by the black, porous walls of these traditional fermenting spaces. The tempeh stays wrapped in banana leaves until the fermentation process is complete and it can be sold at local markets.

Today, genetically modified soybeans from other countries have started finding their way to the island for use in tempeh production. Companies like iniTempe Bali are working to ensure that local soybean farmers on Bali and Java can maintain their farms and help produce tempeh that's local and organic.

Marinated Tempeh

8 ounces tempeh
½ cup water
2 tablespoons olive oil
1 tablespoon of your favorite mustard
1 tablespoon tahini
2 teaspoons maple syrup
2 teaspoons tamari
1 teaspoon fresh lemon juice
Sesame or olive oil, for cooking

Slice the tempeh into strips lengthwise. Slice again in a perpendicular fashion to make cubes.

Throw the tempeh cubes into a large container. Add the water, oil, mustard, tahini, maple syrup, tamari, and lemon juice. Toss with a spoon until the tempeh cubes are well coated.

Set aside in the refrigerator for one hour or up to 24 hours to marinate.

To cook, heat a bit of sesame or olive oil in a skillet over medium heat. Distribute the cubes evenly and brown for 10 minutes on each side. Enjoy as a side dish or add to the recipe below.

🍎 Tempeh with Spinach and Coconut Milk

My host mother taught me how to make this dish when I first visited Bali as a college student, and I continue to prepare it to this day. I am not always able to find galangal, a ginger family rhizome that has a slightly minty flavor, so I sometimes make the recipe without it.

In Bali, my host family and I would walk down to the river, stopping to pray at the elephant god Sri Ganesh's temple and ask permission to harvest the rhizomatic roots of turmeric, ginger, and galangal that grew along the riverbank. I would help pull the plants' tall green fronds aside while my host mother expertly sliced away bright yellow roots in three different shades. She explained to me that the way to know the difference was to compare them: galangal was the pale morning sun, turmeric was the bright midday sun, and ginger was the warm setting sun.

To make this dish, start by marinating the tempeh as described in the recipe above.

As the tempeh marinates, gather the following:

> 2 tablespoons coconut oil
> 2 large shallots, peeled and diced
> 1-inch piece fresh galangal (if you can find it), minced
> 1-inch piece fresh ginger, minced

1-inch piece fresh turmeric, minced, or ½ teaspoon
   ground turmeric

½ teaspoon salt

½ teaspoon garam masala

1 (15-ounce) can unsweetened, full-fat coconut milk

1 large bunch spinach, chopped

Warm the coconut oil in a deep skillet. Add the shallots and the minced galangal (if available), ginger, and turmeric (if using the fresh root) and sauté for 5 minutes, or until the shallots are translucent.

Stir in the salt, garam masala, and ground turmeric (if using the dried root). Add the tempeh and its marinade, along with the coconut milk. Mix gently.

Bring to a boil, then reduce the heat to medium and simmer, with a lid on, for 10 minutes.

Add the spinach to the skillet and simmer for 5 more minutes, until the spinach is well wilted.

Serve with quinoa or rice.

🍎 Ogi

I follow a North African recipe for ogi, millet porridge. I first learned this recipe from Sandor Katz and deepened my understanding of it through linguist Kọ́lá Túbọ̀sún.

My recipe for millet "polenta" as it appears in Katz's book, The Art of Fermentation, *is quite similar to ogi. Both ogi and polenta can be made with either corn or millet, and the similarity between their preparations weaves the traditions of Central America, Africa, and Italy together.*

The "recipe" is really more of a technique:

Soak millet in salted water for 24 hours, then drain it, add more water (three times as much as the millet), and cook it with ground turmeric, ground cumin, ground coriander, salt, and coconut oil. I usually use 1 cup soaked millet, 3 cups water, 2 tablespoons coconut oil, and ½ teaspoon of each of the spices and salt. In the winter, I switch from coconut oil to ghee.

Stir the millet as it cooks until the golden grains melt into a smooth porridge. Pour it into a baking dish and let it set. You can then slice it, toast it, fry it in a skillet, or make it into a thin layer to use as pizza crust. This is a wonderful way to cut down on processed flours and eat more whole grains.

🍎 Quinoa Sourdough Starter

This recipe can be a wonderful alternative to making glutinous bread. As you get comfortable with the process, you can use any grain you like to make the starter and bake bread. Simply get an espresso bean grinder, set it to the fine setting, and grind amaranth, buckwheat, millet, nuts, oats, quinoa, and seeds to make your own flour blends.

> Quinoa flour
> Unchlorinated water
> Raw honey
> Kombucha (optional)
> Flaxseed meal

Mix 1 cup quinoa flour and 1 cup unchlorinated water in a glass quart jar. Add 2 tablespoons raw honey. You can also add a tablespoon of kombucha to expedite fermentation. Cover with a cloth and set it out overnight.

The next day, stir the mixture, then feed it ½ cup quinoa flour and ½ cup water and stir again. Continue to stir throughout the day. Keep it in a warm place. Feed it again the next day and continue stirring periodically. You should start to see some bubbles in the mix. Feed it for 2 more days, continuing to stir and look for bubbles.

Now start feeding it two times a day with quinoa flour and flaxseed meal in a 3-to-1 ratio (¾ cup quinoa flour and ¼ cup flaxseed meal) and 1 cup of water.

Once the starter reaches a volume of about 4 cups, you are ready to make sourdough. Whenever you use it, make sure you leave enough starter to work with for your next batch of bread.

Unless you plan to use the starter every couple of days, you can refrigerate it. When you are ready to make another batch of bread, pull it out of the fridge and feed it for 2 days until it is bubbly and active. Bring it to room temperature before feeding it so that the starter can consume the flour and start to grow.

🍎 Gluten-Free Sourdough Bread

1½ cups quinoa flour (or freshly ground grain flour of your choosing)

1 cup almond flour (or freshly ground nut/seed flour mixture of your choosing)

¾ cup flaxseed meal

3 teaspoons salt

3 cups very active Quinoa Sourdough Starter

1 tablespoon honey or maple syrup

1 cup water or plant milk

Combine the flours, flaxseed meal, and salt in a bowl. Add the starter and honey or maple syrup. Add water or milk ¼ cup at a time, mixing as you go, until you have a smooth, thick batter. This could take up to 5 minutes. Have loved ones take turns if you want to make it a community process.

Line two bread pans with parchment paper, smoothing out any wrinkles. Spoon the dough into the pans and cover them with a thin dish towel. Let the loaves rise for at least 6 hours and up to overnight. The longer they rise, the more sour they will become.

Put the pans in a cold oven and cover them with a baking sheet. Turn the oven temperature to 400°F and bake for 40 minutes. Then uncover the bread pans and bake for 10 minutes more.

Let the loaves set for 30 minutes in their pans, then turn them out onto a cooling rack.

Let the loaves sit for 8 to 12 hours; they will continue to set as time passes. Then feel free to enjoy them.

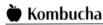 Kombucha

Kombucha is a fermented, lightly carbonated tea beverage offering antimicrobial activity against a range of pathogenic bacteria, thereby promoting immunity and well-being. Its microbial culture, called a SCOBY (symbiotic culture of bacteria and yeast), is a living symbiotic community of yeasts and acetic bacteria that looks like a gelatinous pancake.[10]

The tradition of making kombucha began in ancient China and has traveled through Asia and the Balkans as a digestive strengthener and immune tonic. According to the Merriam-Webster dictionary, the word kombucha seems to be a misinterpretation of the Japanese words konbu, "kelp," and cha, "tea"— perhaps because the SCOBY looks a bit like a mass of seaweed.

The amount of ingredients described here will make a gallon of kombucha, and you'll need a glass gallon jar to hold it. You'll also need a SCOBY, which you can get from a friend who brews kombucha or from the Cultures for Health online store.

> 3 quarts water
> 1 kombucha SCOBY
> 6 tea bags or 6 grams loose-leaf green or black tea
> 1 cup raw honey

Heat the water to boiling. Add the tea (put it in a muslin bag or other steeping material if it's loose leaf). Let steep for the recommended time, which will be dependent on the type of tea you're using. Some people steep their tea for only a few minutes, while others allow it to steep overnight.

Remove the tea. Add the honey and stir to incorporate.

Let the tea cool to room temperature. Then pour it into a glass jar.

Add the kombucha SCOBY to the tea. It may float, sink, or roll onto its side. This is not a problem.

Cover the jar with a tight-knit cloth to prevent pathogens from contaminating the brew. Leave undisturbed in a warm spot (we keep ours on top of the fridge) to ferment for 6 to 8 days.

Enjoy kombucha as flavoring in a glass of water. Drinking a whole glass of it can cause belching, bloating, and gas. A few tablespoons are plenty to gain the probiotic benefit and flavor enhancement.

TRUSTING YOUR GUT

Gut intuition is cultivated over time and becomes clearer as we heal other parts of ourselves. Many cravings come from an imbalance in gut flora as well as depletion of glands in our endocrine system. One of the most common glandular depletions is related to the adrenals. The adrenals are two small glands above the kidneys, and they control a variety of actions, including stress response, weight balance, blood glucose, blood pressure, and immunity, among others.

The adrenal glands control the sympathetic response of the autonomic nervous system—the "fight or flight" state. As described earlier, they release varying amounts of cortisol throughout the day to help us feel more energized in the morning and midday and more tired at night. When the body senses that it is in danger and shifts into sympathetic mode, the adrenals secrete additional cortisol, which releases more glucose into the bloodstream. Once the perceived danger subsides, cortisol levels ideally return to normal, the pancreas secretes insulin to absorb any excess blood glucose, and balance is restored.

However, many people experience a variety of life pressures that push them beyond their limits. When constant pressures place the body in chronic stress mode, the constant adrenal stimulation can cause cortisol to be released at the wrong times of day. This can lead to craving sweets and caffeine to feel alert in the morning and alcohol to wind down in the evening.

Over time, chronic stress causes the adrenals to become taxed. Chinese medicine relates the adrenals to *jing*, or vital essence, and refers to them as the "oil lamps of the soul." These glandular oil lamps can get drawn down and lead to overall depletion. When we lack *jing*, life feels more challenging because the adrenals are not able to tend to acute or chronic stress. Weakened adrenals can lead to symptoms of disease, such as irritability, fatigue, and hypoglycemia.

When this pattern unfolds over time, the body blocks some of its cortisol receptors to restore balance. However, this blockage causes cortisol levels to remain low throughout the day instead of rising and falling as they normally would. This leads to a constant sense of fatigue. Many allopathic doctors refer to this kind of adrenal depletion as "exhaustion syndrome."

Symptoms of adrenal fatigue include:

- Feeling tired and wired at bedtime
- Becoming irritated easily
- Experiencing sugar and carbohydrate cravings
- Feeling tired in the midafternoon
- Gaining abdominal fat

A naturopath or functional medicine doctor can test the adrenals with a cortisol saliva test to start. Further tests measure levels of other hormones, such as DHEA, progesterone, and insulin, to assess the effects of adrenal depletion on the rest of the body.

If you experience a combination of the symptoms above, you can start supporting yourself with relaxation techniques such as breathwork, mindful eating, gentle movement, and protein-based meals. These strategies support the body in restoring adrenal balance.

Meal Plan for Adrenal Balance

Breakfast: 2 eggs scrambled with spinach, salt, and olive oil; 1 cup roasted sweet potatoes drizzled with flaxseed oil

Lunch: 4 ounces cooked chicken breast; 1 cup steamed asparagus mixed with with 2 tablespoons ghee and 1 cup cooked quinoa

Dinner: 4 ounces cooked salmon; 1½ cups steamed broccoli garnished with homemade aioli; 1 cup wild rice

Snacks: seaweed snacks with ¼ cup almonds; 1 cup oatmeal with ¼ cup blueberries, 2 tablespoons coconut oil, and 2 tablespoons flaxseed meal; 1 cup chia pudding

LESSONS FROM AYAHUASCA

Ultimately, trusting the gut is a practice developed over time that harnesses the power of intuition. While I was healing from chronic infection, I began to see the benefits of the traditional foods and herbs I was using. Through conversations with friends who were on their own healing journey, I learned about an indigenous brew from the Amazon known as *ayahuasca, natém, nixi pãe,* and *yahé,* among other names. This brew is made from the vines of an Amazonian plant (Latin name *Banisteriopsis caapi*) as well as other ingredients, which are specific to the role desired by each tribe that brews them. Ayahuasca has been used ritually for visionary and healing purposes for more than five thousand years. It is proprietary to indigenous tribes of the Amazon. Yubaka Hayrá, the first gathering of indigenous ayahuasca practitioners, took place in Brazil in 2017. Representatives from many Amazonian tribes as well as Brazilian spiritual groups such as Santo Daime, Barquinha, and União do Vegetal were in attendance. This conference, "jointly emphasized the responsibility of indigenous peoples, as the original recipients and bearers of the medicine, to preserve scientific and spiritual knowledge."[11]

Being in right relationship with this sacred medicine means honoring the people who created it and using it in accordance with their requests. I had the great privilege of traveling to Ecuador and engaging in ceremony with a healer from the Shuar tribe. This healer is extremely experienced in working with ayahuasca for physical healing purposes; the Shuar are a warrior tribe and prize physical health.

When I met this healer and told him about my parasitic infection, he immediately identified me as someone who had done *emasiado drogas,* "too many drugs." He was not wrong: as a teen, I found that the mind-altering experience offered by plants such as psilocybin and cannabis distracted me from the pain of assimilation. I understood his reflection as a reminder that, when someone is too open spiritually and imbalanced con-stitutionally by something like overuse of consciousness-shifting plants, it is easier for a pathogen such as a parasite to become chronic in their body.

After the first all-night healing ceremony we did in Ecuador, I felt so depleted that I wanted to give up and go home. We had listened to stories, prayed over the medicine, taken the medicine, received a treat-ment from the healer, drunk herbs that caused purging, done enemas, and prayed more. Although I do not consciously remember, everyone present was stunned by my body's thrashing and the sounds that came out of me during my treatment. Not only were the antibiotic com-pounds in the medicine eradicating parasites, but the healer was draw-ing out the spiritual invasion caused by my lack of energetic boundaries.

That first ceremony felt like a dispossession, and I was both physically and spiritually exhausted from it. Not to mention that I weighed about ninety pounds at that time (and I am five feet, six inches tall) and we could not eat past noon in preparation for each ceremony. It had taken me a year to build up the courage to leave my house and travel on a plane to a place where I had no control over my food or environment. When I told my friends how I was feeling, they took me back to the healer's house. He began to sing a silly song with the words "Lisa tiene miedo," meaning "Lisa is scared." Once again, he nailed it. I was terrified. I feared the unknown and the transformative quality of this profound healing process. By the time he was done singing, we had all joined in and I was laughing so much that tears streamed down my face. After that, I was ready for another ceremony.

And so it continued for three more weeks. When we would eat a hearty meal the morning after a ceremony, my gut intuition was suddenly available again. We would purchase food at the market, I would hold my hand over it, close my eyes, take a deep breath, and thank it for all it had to offer. Then I would eat. If I ever got a message that a food was not ideal in that moment, I would skip it and try it again the following day. Trust had replaced fear. My enteric nervous system was able to relax so that my body could digest the food I was eating. From avocados and pasta to corn and *papacinas* (indigenous potatoes), I rediscovered the feeling I had experienced at the silent meditation retreat: when I was calm and centered, I could offer gratitude for a meal and my body could digest food and assimilate nutrients.

When I returned to Vermont, this renewed sense of fortitude remained with me. Ayahuasca acted as a plant antibiotic to combat my infection while allowing my gut to maintain a balance of the beneficial bacteria I needed to heal. The indigenous healer with whom we worked offered the spiritual support and nervous system reset that I needed to trust the unfolding of my healing process. As my health started to improve, I gathered friends together to help me call back my menstrual cycle, which had been absent for six years. I worked with a somatic movement teacher to process the trauma that comes with chronic illness. I continued to include more and more foods in my daily eating and started crafting recipes to rebuild my body. I never could have imagined that I would heal to the point where I could conceive and give birth. When I look at my two children today, I know that they represent the body's infinite capacity to heal.

Modern medicine can be a blessing in an emergency or after other approaches have not been successful. However, the body has infinite capacity to heal; plants and foods have coevolved with humans to support that healing process. As Wendell Berry wrote in *Sex, Economy, Freedom & Community: Eight Essays*, "People are fed by the food industry, which pays no attention to health, and are treated by the health industry, which pays no attention to food." As we return to the guidance of intuition, may we all have the ability to access whole, traditional foods for nourishment and healing so that the food and health industries no longer play their current roles in society.

6

Nutrients and Wellness

Food Types and Combinations

*Not so long ago, there were people who had true virtue,
understood the way of life, and were able to adapt to and
harmonize with the universe and the seasons.*

THE YELLOW EMPEROR'S CLASSIC OF MEDICINE
(THIRD MILLENNIUM BCE)

Centuries-old Chinese medicine texts understood that health is founded in connection with the surrounding environment. Humans connect with nature by taking it in, both physically through eating and experientially through living in a landscape. Adaptation is essential to survival, and the plants with which people have coevolved are necessary for life. Through multiple healing journeys, I have learned that traditional healing systems worldwide already knew centuries ago what nutritionists learn today. Nutritionists talk about macronutrients (carbohydrates, protein, fat, water) and micronutrients (vitamins and minerals). Traditional foodways explain the same concepts about nutrient balance by discussing seasonal eating, the importance of plants as nourishment, and balancing meals by including all the flavors.

When we are trying to understand what a nutrition plan customized for our own unique needs might look like, it can be helpful to consider the role of the various nutrients the body uses to thrive. Macronutrients ("big" nutrients) and micronutrients ("small" nutrients) are crucial to human survival. Their ideal balance is different for everyone, depending on many factors. Macronutrients include carbohydrates, protein, and fat. The more whole foods we eat, the more micronutrients are included in our macronutrient intake. We get more vitamins and minerals from a sweet potato, for example, than from crackers.

CARBOHYDRATES

Carbohydrates provide energy for both the body and the brain. They also help the body process fat, breaking it down into fatty acids. The fiber in carbohydrates ensures smooth transit of food through the digestive tract. When we consume carbohydrates, the digestive system converts them into glucose, which the body uses as energy for cells, tissues, and organs. How many carbohydrates does an individual need? This depends on factors such as activity level, age, preference, and genetic background.

Simple Carbohydrates

Our ancestors who were hunter-gatherers rarely encountered short-chain, or simple, carbohydrates. Yet today they are abundant in the food system. Large-scale food manufacturers have created an industry that profits from generating addiction to highly processed foods that are far from their original form. Ingesting simple carbohydrates leads to a rapid and steep rise in both blood glucose and insulin levels. About one and a half to two hours after consuming simple carbohydrates, the body feels hungry again—a feeling that can only be satisfied by consuming more simple carbohydrates.

It can be helpful to pair simple carbohydrates with fat, which helps the body metabolize them, and protein, which slows their metabolism. This way, the body feels fuller for longer. Sources of simple carbohydrates that are less processed and thus less challenging for the body to digest include:

Raw honey: rich in calcium, iron, magnesium, niacin, pantothenic acid, phosphorus, potassium, riboflavin, selenium, thiamin, vitamin B_6, and zinc

Maple syrup: rich in antioxidants, calcium, iron, magnesium, manganese, potassium, prebiotics, probiotics, and zinc

Molasses: rich in calcium, iron, magnesium, selenium, and vitamin B_6

Fresh fruit and vegetable juices: high in antioxidants, minerals, and vitamins

Complex Carbohydrates

Complex carbohydrates are composed of three or more sugars. They contain fiber, vitamins, and minerals. They take longer to digest than simple carbohydrates, so they don't raise blood glucose as quickly. Instead, they provide fuel for longer periods and help mitochondria produce energy. Vegetables and whole grains are examples of complex carbohydrates. While most complex carbohydrates are digested slowly, some are higher on the glycemic index and could lead to elevated blood glucose. Flours tend to place a higher glycemic load on the body than whole grains, for example.

Unrefined whole grains are rich in vitamins, minerals, and fiber. But depending on our genetics, grains may increase insulin levels and interfere with the body's capacity to burn fat. As we get to know our bodies, we better understand which foods are ideal for our unique constitution. If our cholesterol level or blood pressure is elevated or if insulin resistance is a factor, decreasing consumption of grains and simple carbohydrates for a period of time can help the body to regain balance.

There are two types of complex carbohydrates: oligosaccharides and polysaccharides. Oligosaccharides support immune function, help the body absorb minerals, facilitate digestive transit time, and form fatty acids. Oligosaccharides are also prebiotics; they feed beneficial gut bacteria. Oligosaccharides can be found in asparagus, burdock, chicory, chives, garlic, green bananas, Jerusalem artichokes, leeks, and onions, among others. (If any of these foods feels hard to digest, it is time to take a look at gut flora and nourish it with a specific strain of probiotic that helps break down oligosaccharides; see chapter 5.)

Polysaccharides are the most complex type of carbohydrate. They need to be thoroughly digested before they can be absorbed. There are two categories of polysaccharides: starches and nonstarches. Nonstarch polysaccharides support healthy blood sugar and cholesterol levels, soothe the joints and intestinal lining, and support healthy immunity. They can be found in aloe, flaxseed, mushrooms, and seaweed. Starchy polysaccharides turn into glucose that the body can use both as energy and to feed beneficial gut bacteria. They can be found in beans, brown rice, lentils, oats, potatoes, quinoa, sweet potatoes, winter squash, and yams, among others.

If you are craving certain carbohydrates, pay attention to whether they are simple or complex and starchy or not. This will allow you to follow your intuition as to what to eat and why you are having a specific craving. Craving complex carbohydrates is your body's way of asking for sustainable fuel. Craving simple carbohydrates may be more related to needing short-term fuel, being thirsty, or feeling tired.

Fiber
Although it is technically part of the carbohydrate category, fiber deserves special attention because the body can become unbalanced when it gets either too much or not enough fiber. Proper fiber consumption is a fine balance that varies based on constitution, age, and environment.

Fiber comes exclusively from plants. We need both the soluble (viscous) type and the insoluble (bulking) type. Soluble fiber dissolves into a mucilage, which helps capture and eliminate toxins and cholesterol from the body. Insoluble fiber is not digested by the body or absorbed into the bloodstream. Instead, it forms most stools in the body, acting as an intestinal sweeper. Both forms can help us feel full by creating volume in the digestive tract that lets the brain know the body is nourished. Each kind also has specific benefits that are tied to how the body handles them.

Soluble Fiber

Soluble fiber dissolves in water and slows the speed at which carbohydrates are absorbed in the body. This helps prevent blood glucose spikes and reduces the chances of feeling irritable or developing insulin resistance. Soluble fiber also supports heart health and reduces the risk of heart disease by balancing cholesterol levels.

Certain soluble fibers are fermentable. When they reach the large intestine, gut bacteria feed on them, creating short-chain fatty acids (SCFAs) like butyrate, acetate, and propionate. These SCFAs can provide energy, improve metabolism, regulate blood sugar levels, and reduce chronic inflammation. However, too much fermentable fiber can cause bloating, gas, and cramping in the large intestine, especially if our microbiome is out of balance. If you experience these symptoms after eating foods rich in soluble fiber, consider a test like a complete metabolic panel to get a better understanding of which nutrients you digest and which ones are harder for your body to break down.

Foods that are high in soluble fiber tend to also be rich in starchy polysaccharides. They include apricots, beans, blueberries, broccoli, Brussels sprouts, carrots, figs, flaxseed, lentils, oats, sweet potatoes, and turnips.

Insoluble Fiber

Insoluble fiber doesn't dissolve in water and passes through the digestive system intact, giving it a more laxative effect. When insoluble fiber moves through the digestive tract, it pulls water into the stool, making it softer and easier to pass. This can help alleviate constipation and improve digestive function. Although more research has to be done on the role of soluble fiber in body weight reduction, insoluble fiber may help you maintain balanced weight. Starting the day with a breakfast high in insoluble fiber accelerates your metabolic rate and helps the body feel satiated until lunchtime. Since insoluble fiber doesn't get broken down by the body, it has no effect on blood glucose.

Foods that are high in insoluble fiber include amaranth, arugula, avocado, brown rice, cauliflower, chia seeds, kale, pumpkin seeds, and spinach.

♥ Amaranth Porridge

For the Aztec, amaranth was not only a dietary staple but an important aspect of religious rituals. Although amaranth derives its name from the Greek word for never-fading flower, it is the highly nutritious seeds (and greens, though they are hard to find), not the vibrant red blooms, that are most nutrient dense. Like buckwheat and quinoa, amaranth is both gluten-free and rich in plant proteins, including two essential amino acids, lysine and methionine. It has a nutty, slightly bitter flavor.

1 tablespoon olive oil or coconut oil

¼ teaspoon salt

¼ teaspoon ground cinnamon

¼ teaspoon ground coriander

4 cups water or coconut milk

1 cup amaranth

1 cup quinoa

½ teaspoon apple cider vinegar or fresh lemon juice

¼ cup hemp seeds

Place all the ingredients except the hemp seeds in a pot. Bring to a boil, then reduce the heat and let simmer for 25 minutes, or until the porridge begins to thicken. Stir occasionally to make sure it is not sticking to the bottom.

Mix in the hemp seeds and enjoy.

FATS

The three main forms of fat found in food are triglycerides, phospholipids, and sterols, primarily in the form of cholesterol. These nutrients provide about nine calories per gram of energy, compared with four calories per gram from carbohydrates and proteins. Fats are not absorbed directly by any tissue. Instead, they must be hydrolyzed outside the cells into fatty acids and glycerol, which can then enter cells. In other words, to metabolize fats, the body must use energy, primarily from carbohydrates in glucose form, to produce energy.

The two sources of fat we use in our body are food (both from fats and certain proteins) and adipocytes (the body's fat cells). Food sources of fats include nuts, seeds, oils, dairy, and certain meats and fish. In addition to the protein (amino acid) content of meat and fish, some contain fats. Beef, lamb, certain cuts of pork, chicken skin, and salmon are examples of proteins that contain fats.

Adipocytes, or adipose tissue in the body, are not only important for survival but they are also an endocrine gland that secretes hormones. In utero, first blood vessels and nerve cells form, and then fat tissue forms. The organ that holds the digestive tract and other organs together is called the mesentery. From the Greek meaning "middle intestine," this fat-based organ is the container in which the digestive system develops in a fetus. It has blood vessels, neurotransmitters, and lymph ducts and nodules. Without the mesentery, digestion and immunity would not function properly. Fat is essential to life.

Fat from food, adipocytes (fat cells), and amino acids is broken down in the mitochondria of the cells and then synthesized in the liver, adipose tissue, and intestinal mucosa. The fatty acids derived from this process are essential for metabolizing carbohydrates and using them as energy.

Among other vital functions, fats:

- Maintain body temperature and insulation
- Provide protective padding for internal organs and nerves
- Maintain a healthy nervous system response
- Reduce oxidative stress that leads to chronic inflammation
- Stimulate the secretion of bile salts for digestion and the absorption of fat-soluble vitamins (A, D, E, and K)
- Support the structure and integrity of cell membranes
- Maintain cell regulatory signals (essential to combating autoimmune conditions)
- Help balance hormonal function
- Keep the skin supple
- Provide flavor and satiety

When the body does not have enough fats provided to it, it begins to store carbohydrates as fat because it does not know when it will next gain this essential nutrient. Hence, when the body is deprived of fat, it may crave carbohydrates. When we consume healthy fats, on the other hand, the body feels satisfied with less food; the brain releases endorphins to signal fullness, relax, and lubricate the digestive system so that it can effectively process carbohydrates and proteins.

We support strength and ease in the body by eating high-quality fats, such as olive, sunflower, and coconut oils; animal fats from poultry, eggs, and fish; and hormone-free butter.[1] (Animal fats are not necessary, of course; the choice is yours.)

Saturated versus Unsaturated

Fats are made up of chains of fatty acids. Whether a fat is saturated or unsaturated depends on the number of double bonds in the chain and the length of the chain. Saturated fats have no double bonds, making them more stable and solid at room temperature. Saturated fats include those found in animal products, such as dairy products and fatty meats, and certain vegetable oils, including coconut and palm kernel oil. Several studies have shown that saturated fats can trigger adipose fat inflammation, an indicator of heart disease and worsening of arthritis inflammation. Unsaturated fats have one (monounsaturated) or more (polyunsaturated) bonds. Vegetable oils are the most abundant sources of unsaturated fats. Having the right balance of saturated and unsaturated fats is important for preventing inflammation.

The polyunsaturated omega-3 fatty acids, found in flax, borage, and evening primrose oils as well as salmon, cod, and sardines, have tremendous health benefits. Among other things, they help reduce inflammation, maintain cell membrane fluidity, lower the amount of lipids (fats such as cholesterol and triglycerides) in the bloodstream, decrease platelet aggregation (preventing excessive blood clotting), and reduce the production of cytokines, which are involved in the inflammatory response of atherosclerosis. Omega-3s also improve the body's ability to respond to insulin by stimulating the secretion of leptin, a hormone that helps us know when we are satiated after eating a meal.

Omega-6 fatty acids are essential for normal growth and development. However, when eaten in excess, they can trigger the body to produce pro-inflammatory chemicals. These fatty acids are found in high levels in many polyunsaturated oils such as corn, safflower, sunflower, grapeseed, soy, peanut, and vegetable oil blends, as well as mayonnaise and many commercial salad dressings. An optimal balance or ratio of omega-6 to omega-3 fatty acids is 2:1 or 3:1. Eating more foods rich in omega-3 fatty acids is a useful strategy for maintaining health.

Cholesterol

As with fiber, cholesterol deserves a bit of extra attention because the medical community is hyperfocused on it. Cholesterol is a sterol, a type of lipid the body can both create and get from food. The body is excellent at striking the balance between what we take in through eating and what it produces in the liver. When we eat more cholesterol, the body produces less; when we eat less cholesterol, the body produces more. Foods from both plants and animals contain sterols, but only animal products contain cholesterol. Cholesterol is part of nearly every cell and supports cellular integrity. It is a precursor of estrogen, testosterone, cortisol, and vitamin D. Approximately 25 percent of the brain is comprised of cholesterol. Myelin sheaths that insulate nerve cells and in the synapses that transmit nerve impulses are made primarily of cholesterol. It also supports the uptake of hormones in the brain, including serotonin.

LDL versus HDL

When the body sustains an injury, inflammation triggers the liver to release cholesterol into the blood to help create a scar. This kind of cholesterol is called low-density lipoprotein (LDL). When the body is in a state of chronic inflammation, LDL cholesterol works to help repair cellular damage, which leads to higher amounts of cholesterol in the blood than the body can manage. It can thicken and become plaque, thereby decreasing blood flow and causing blood pressure to increase so that blood can keep moving through the restricted channels.

High-density lipoprotein (HDL) cholesterol can move LDL cholesterol from artery walls and discard it, with the liver's assistance. High levels of LDL cholesterol and low levels of HDL cholesterol are risk factors for atherosclerosis, which is arterial congestion. For optimal cardiovascular health, the American Heart Association recommends LDL blood levels of less than 100 mg/dL and HDL blood levels of greater than 60 mg/dL.

Achieving Healthy Cholesterol

HDL is sometimes called "good" cholesterol and LDL "bad" cholesterol. In truth, neither is good nor bad. We simply need a balance between them. The foods we eat, genetics, and lifestyle are what determine the way the body transports and deposits fats—though studies have shown that genetics have more of an impact on the body's cholesterol balance than food does.[2]

What are ways to attain and maintain cholesterol balance? To begin, when we eat more plant foods and move our bodies, HDL cholesterol has more tools to keep shuttling accumulations of LDL cholesterol out of the body. We can avoid refined carbohydrates, which, depending on genetics, can interfere with the body's ability to burn fat, thus leading to cholesterol imbalance. Nonstarchy polysaccharides, like those found in seaweed, flaxseed meal, and mushrooms, can help the body naturally balance cholesterol levels. Soluble fiber can do the same, so enjoy oatmeal and oat bran, chia seeds, beans, lentils, peas, and pectin-rich foods such as apples, strawberries, and citrus fruit.

Omega-3 fatty acids are crucial to cholesterol balance. Conjugated linoleic acid (CLA) in particular has shown beneficial effects in supporting healthy cholesterol ratios.[3] Beef and butter from grass-fed cows are high in CLA, as are unpasteurized goat and sheep dairy products.

Sound counterintuitive? Well, that's because the medical community looks at symptoms, not root causes. Moderate amounts of high-CLA foods are essential to establishing balanced lipid metabolism and cholesterol levels. Aim for high-CLA foods to be about 10 percent of your daily fat intake.

Taking two tablespoons of food-grade aloe vera gel before bed can help the body metabolize fat and therefore balance overall cholesterol levels.

The Dangers of Statins

Statins are cholesterol-lowering drugs, and they are among the most widely prescribed drugs in the United States. Ultimately, statins interfere with the body's ability to produce cholesterol, therefore reducing the amount of cholesterol available for the body to use. Side effects of statins include liver damage, muscle wasting, increased blood glucose, memory loss, depletion of vitamin K and coenzyme Q_{10}, disrupted production of hormones (especially serotonin and reproductive hormones), and mental imbalance.

To optimize cholesterol, try to stay away from statins. Instead, eliminate refined sugars from your eating, because when insulin is balanced, HDL cholesterol can do its shuttling work much more effectively. Try including anti-inflammatory foods such as leafy greens, olive oil, coconut oil, pastured eggs, avocados, flaxseed, and grass-fed meats in your meals.

PROTEINS

Proteins are made of small units called amino acids. In various forms, proteins help build muscle, assist in immune defense, heal wounds, and make up collagen, the connective tissue that tones the body and skin.

All enzymes are proteins, and they serve as catalysts to chemical reactions in the body. Among other things, they support the functioning of the liver, stomach, and blood and help convert glycogen to glucose for energy. Examples include the enzymes amylase, which helps digest carbohydrates, and protease, which breaks down protein. If necessary, the liver can convert amino acids from protein into glucose through a process called gluconeogenesis.

The digestion of protein in the stomach begins with pepsins, which break down protein into smaller peptides. Further along, in the small intestine, trypsin and chymotrypsin continue this process with the help of microvilli—small, fingerlike structures that increase the absorptive surface area of the small intestine. Once protein is broken down into its amino acid components, the amino acids can be absorbed from the intestines into the bloodstream.

Amino Acids

Amino acids that can't be manufactured in the body and must be obtained through food are referred to as essential. The essential amino acids are histidine, isoleucine, leucine, lysine, methionine, phenylalanine, threonine, tryptophan, and valine. Amino acids that can be made by our body are referred to as nonessential. The nonessential amino acids are alanine, arginine, asparagine, aspartic acid, cysteine, glutamic acid, glutamine, glycine, proline, serine, and tyrosine.

Certain nonessential amino acids are sometimes called "conditionally essential" because they can be synthesized in the body from other amino acids. The conditionally essential amino acids are arginine, cysteine, glutamine, glycine, proline, serine, and tyrosine.

Functions of Essential Amino Acids

- **Histidine** aids in the production of red and white blood cells and can be used to treat anemia. It can also be helpful in reversing autoimmune conditions, specifically rheumatoid arthritis. It is one of the skin's ultraviolet-absorbing compounds.
- **Isoleucine** is quick fuel for muscles. It is helpful in preventing muscle wasting and essential to the formation of hemoglobin.
- **Leucine** helps reduce muscle protein breakdown and promotes the healing of skin and broken bones.

- **Lysine** inhibits viruses and is used in the treatment of the herpes simplex virus (HSV). Lysine and vitamin C together form L-carnitine, a biochemical that enables muscle to use oxygen more efficiently. Lysine aids bone growth by helping form collagen, the fibrous protein that makes up bone, cartilage, and other connective tissue.

- **Methionine** is a precursor of cysteine and creatine. It helps increase antioxidant levels and reduces blood cholesterol levels. It removes waste from the liver and assists in the regeneration of liver and kidney tissue.

- **Phenylalanine** is the primary precursor of tyrosine. It enhances learning, memory, and mood.

- **Threonine** helps immune cells eradicate infection. The nervous system uses threonine to make glycine. It is found in high concentrations in the heart, skeletal muscles, and central nervous system. Threonine supports the functioning of the liver, nervous system, and cardiovascular system.

- **Tryptophan** is a precursor of the relaxation hormone serotonin. It stimulates the release of growth hormones and is popularly known for its prevalence in turkey meat.

- **Valine** bypasses the liver so that it can be used immediately by the muscles. It supports the brain in taking up tryptophan, phenylalanine, and tyrosine.

Functions of Nonessential Amino Acids

- **Alanine** is a component of connective tissue and helps muscles and other tissues gain fuel from other amino acids. It also helps restore immune system strength after illness.

- **Arginine** can increase insulin, glucagon, and growth hormone levels. It aids in the formation of collagen. It is a precursor of creatine and gamma-aminobutyric acid (GABA), a neurotransmitter in the brain.

- **Asparagine** fights fatigue and helps the liver function properly.

- **Aspartic acid** helps convert carbohydrates into energy. It builds immune system immunoglobulins and antibodies and reduces ammonia levels after exercise.
- **Cysteine** contributes to strong connective tissue and tissue antioxidant actions. It aids in healing, stimulates white blood cells, and helps reduce pain. It helps form skin and hair.
- **Glutamic acid**, which the body synthesizes into glutamine, is a non-essential amino acid that functions as a neurotransmitter and supports healthy nervous system function, particularly in the brain.
- **Glutamine** is the most abundant amino acid in the body. It plays a key role in immune system function, provides energy to the kidneys, heals tears in the intestinal lining (leaky gut syndrome), fuels the brain, and supports concentration.
- **Glycine** aids in manufacturing other amino acids and is a part of the structure of hemoglobin and cytochromes (enzymes involved in energy production). It has a calming effect and is sometimes used to support recovery from mental imbalance.
- **Proline** helps form connective tissue and heart muscle. It is readily mobilized for muscular energy and is a major constituent of collagen.
- **Serine** is important in cells' energy production. It aids memory and nervous system function. It helps strengthen the immune system by producing immunoglobulins and antibodies.
- **Tyrosine** is a precursor to dopamine, norepinephrine, and epinephrine, as well as thyroid hormones, growth hormones, and melanin, the pigment responsible for skin and hair color. It can help balance mild depression.

Vegan Protein

Veganism is the practice of abstaining from the use of animal products and an associated philosophy that rejects the commodity status of animals. Distinctions may be made between several categories of veganism. Dietary vegans, also known as "strict vegetarians," refrain from consuming meat, eggs, dairy products, and any other animal-derived substances.

Dorothy Morgan and Donald Watson are said to have coined the term *vegan* in 1944 when they cofounded the Vegan Society in the United Kingdom. At first, they used it to mean vegetarians who do not eat dairy products. However, by May 1945, vegans explicitly abstained from any foods that were sourced from animals, including eggs and honey. In the late 1940s Leslie J. Cross offered the first definition of veganism as "the principle of emancipation of animals from exploitation of man."[4] Interest in veganism increased in the 2010s, especially in the latter half, with more vegan stores opening and more vegan options becoming increasingly available in supermarkets and restaurants.

For those who do not eat animal-derived foods, it is important to consider how to obtain complete proteins. There are a few plant foods that contain all nine essential amino acids, including buckwheat, chia seeds, hemp seeds, and spirulina. Other foods, such as nuts, seeds, beans, lentils, and grains, are rich in protein but are considered incomplete because they are missing one or more of the essential amino acids. This is when pairing foods comes in handy. For example, beans are a great source for the amino acid lysine but are low in methionine. Rice, on the other hand, is low in lysine but a great source for methionine. When you put beans and rice together, you have a complete protein.

With intention, vegetarians and vegans can consume enough protein in their meals to feel vibrant and energized. But note that those on a vegan diet will need to supplement with vitamin B_{12}, which is found only in animal-derived foods.

Plant-Based Complete Proteins
Almonds: 9 grams complete protein per ¼ cup
Buckwheat: 7 grams complete protein per 1 cup
Cashews: 7 grams complete protein per ¼ cup
Chia seeds: 6 grams complete protein per ¼ cup
Flax seeds: 10 grams complete protein per ¼ cup
Hemp seeds: 12 grams complete protein per ¼ cup

Macadamia nuts: 12 grams complete protein per ¼ cup

¼ cup nut butter + 2 slices sourdough wheat bread: 15 grams
complete protein

Pecans: 11 grams complete protein per ¼ cup

Quinoa: 8 grams complete protein per 1 cup

Rice and beans: 8 grams complete protein per 1 cup (½ cup of each)

Tempeh: 15 grams complete protein per ½ cup

♥ Macadamia Nut Sauce

    1 cup macadamia nuts (or cashews)
    3 tablespoons nutritional yeast
    2 cloves garlic
    ½ teaspoon salt
    1 tablespoon fresh lemon juice
    ¼ cup olive oil
    ¼ cup water

Combine all the ingredients in a blender and blend together.

Try spreading this sauce on a Farinata Pizza crust (see page 51)
after you've baked it for the first 15 minutes. Top with vegetables,
such as mushrooms, spinach, basil, and artichokes, and bake as
directed in that recipe.

♥ Kasha Biscuits

    1 cup kasha
    2½ cups water
    ¼ cup olive oil
    2 tablespoons flaxseed meal
    ¼ teaspoon ground nutmeg
    ¼ teaspoon salt
    Juice and zest of 1 lemon

Combine the kasha and water in a stock pot. Bring to a boil,
then reduce the heat and simmer, uncovered, for 15 minutes, or
until the kasha begins to thicken.

Stir the kasha vigorously until it reaches a porridge-like consistency. Set aside to cool for 15 minutes.

Meanwhile, preheat the oven to 375°F. Grease a baking dish.

In a bowl, mix the olive oil, flaxseed, nutmeg, and salt. Stir in the cooled kasha and then the lemon juice and zest.

Drop the mixture in heaping spoonfuls on a greased baking dish. Bake for 15 minutes, or until the edges have turned dark brown. Let cool for 15 minutes before serving.

♥ Herbed Green Gravy

2 tablespoons olive oil

1 medium yellow onion, diced

2 cloves garlic, minced

1½ teaspoons dried rosemary

1½ teaspoons dried thyme

¼ teaspoon salt

½ teaspoon freshly ground black pepper

¼ cup arrowroot flour

2 cups vegetable broth

2 cups chopped dark leafy greens

Heat the oil in a medium pot over medium heat. Add the onion and cook until softened and translucent, about 5 minutes, stirring frequently.

Add the garlic, rosemary, thyme, salt, and pepper. Add the flour and stir until a paste forms. Let cook for about 1 minute.

Add a few splashes of the broth. Let cook for 2 minutes, then pour in the rest of the broth. Whisk until well combined.

Add the greens. Bring to a boil, uncovered, stirring occasionally. Once the gravy is boiling, reduce the heat and simmer for about 10 minutes.

Remove from the heat and let sit for about 10 minutes to thicken more. Stir before serving. For smooth gravy, pour the mixture into a blender and blend.

Serve over Kasha Biscuits (page 139).

❤ Santa Fe-Style Scramble

I learned this recipe from my favorite vegetarian restaurant in Santa Fe, New Mexico. The restaurant used northern New Mexican red chiles, but I use red bell peppers because those chiles are harder to find and are registered as protected through Slow Food's Ark of Taste.

> 8 ounces tempeh
> ½ teaspoon ground cumin
> ½ teaspoon ground turmeric
> ¼ teaspoon chili powder
> Salt and freshly ground black pepper
> Olive oil
> I red onion, chopped
> I red pepper, chopped
> 2 cups kale, loosely chopped

Chop the tempeh into cubes. Bring a small pot of water to a boil, add the tempeh cubes, and simmer them for 10 minutes.

Meanwhile, prepare the sauce: Combine the cumin, turmeric, chili powder, and ½ teaspoon salt in a small bowl. Whisk in enough water to make a pourable sauce. Set aside.

Warm a large skillet over medium heat. Once it is hot, add I to 2 tablespoons olive oil, followed by the onion and red pepper. Season with a pinch of salt and pepper and stir. Cook until softened, about 5 minutes.

Add the kale, season with a bit more salt and pepper, and cover to steam for 2 minutes.

Make a well in the center of the skillet and add the tempeh cubes. Sauté for 2 minutes, then add the sauce, pouring it mostly over the tempeh and a little over the veggies.

Stir well, cook for 5 minutes more, then serve and enjoy.

♥ Tagine-Inspired Stew

Tagine is the name of both the earthenware pot in which this dish is traditionally cooked and the dish itself. Records of this dish date back to the ninth century in North Africa.

    3 tablespoons coconut oil
    1 onion, chopped
    3 cups vegetable broth
    ½ teaspoon ground coriander
    ½ teaspoon ground cumin
    ¼ teaspoon ground black pepper
    ¼ teaspoon ground cinnamon
    ¼ teaspoon ground fenugreek
    ¼ teaspoon salt
    1 large sweet potato (about 1 pound), peeled and cut
        into ½-inch pieces
    1-inch piece of kombu or wakame seaweed, chopped
    1 tablespoon fresh lemon juice
    1 cup cooked chickpeas

Heat the oil in a stock pot. Add the onion and sauté briefly.

Stir in ⅓ cup of the broth and cook for 5 minutes longer.

Stir in the spices and salt. Cook for 1 minute, stirring. Add the remaining 2⅔ cups broth, along with the sweet potato, seaweed, and lemon juice.

Bring to a boil over medium-high heat, then reduce the heat to low, cover, and simmer for about 20 minutes, or until the sweet potato is tender. Add the chickpeas, heat through, and enjoy.

♥ Shepherd's Pie

For the filling:

    2 tablespoons olive oil, plus a bit for oiling the pie plate
    1 large carrot, chopped
    2 cloves garlic, minced
    ½ teaspoon salt

½ teaspoon freshly ground black pepper

½ teaspoon ground coriander

½ teaspoon ground cumin

½ teaspoon dried thyme

1 cup cooked pinto beans

1 cup fresh or frozen peas

For the topping:

½ cup red potatoes

1 cup cooked winter squash or sweet potatoes

¼ cup water

¼ teaspoon salt

2 tablespoons olive oil

Start with the potatoes for the topping: Chop the red potatoes. Boil them in water until tender. Drain, saving some of the cooking water for blending them. Set aside.

Make the filling: Heat a skillet over medium-high heat. Add the olive oil, followed by the carrots. Sauté until the carrots start to brown. Then add the garlic, salt, and spices and stir together. Add the beans and peas and let cook for a few more minutes. Then turn off the heat.

Preheat the oven to 400°F. Oil a pie plate with olive oil.

Place cooked potatoes, cooked squash or sweet potatoes, water, oil, and salt in blender and blend until smooth (or blend with an immersion blender).

Spread the vegetable sauté in the pie plate. Top with the potato mixture, spreading it out evenly.

Bake for 15 minutes, or until the topping is starting to brown. You can broil the dish for a few moments at the end of the baking time if you like the topping to be crispier.

Remove from the oven and let cool for 10 minutes before eating.

♥ Zucchini Bake

4 medium zucchini

2 tablespoons olive oil, plus a bit for oiling the baking sheet

I large onion, sliced

3 cups sliced mushrooms

I teaspoon apple cider vinegar

½ cup vegetable broth

I cup macadamia nuts

I clove garlic, minced

I tablespoon nutritional yeast

I tablespoon mustard of choice

¼ teaspoon ground nutmeg

¼ teaspoon salt

½ cup water

Additional salt and freshly ground black pepper to taste

Preheat the oven to 400°F. Oil a baking sheet with olive oil.

Slice the zucchini into rounds, sprinkle with salt and pepper, and lay out in a single layer on baking sheet.

Bake for 25 minutes.

Meanwhile, heat the olive oil in a deep skillet. Add the onion, salt and pepper to taste, and sauté for 10 minutes over medium-low heat, until the onion is golden. Add the mushrooms, vinegar, and broth and cook over low heat, covered, for 15 minutes. Stir occasionally.

Meanwhile, make the sauce: Combine the macadamias, garlic, nutritional yeast, mustard, nutmeg, salt, and water in in a blender or food processor and process until smooth.

Remove the zucchini from oven and add to skillet with onions and mushrooms. Mix well. Serve the vegetables over quinoa or rice, topped with the macadamia sauce.

❦ Red Lentil Chili

> 2 tablespoons olive oil
>
> 1 white or yellow onion, diced
>
> 1 red bell pepper, diced
>
> ½ teaspoon salt
>
> ½ teaspoon freshly ground black pepper
>
> 4 cloves garlic, minced
>
> 1 teaspoon ground coriander
>
> 1 teaspoon ground cumin
>
> 1 teaspoon paprika
>
> ½ teaspoon chili powder
>
> 2 cups homemade or canned organic pumpkin puree
>
> 2 cups vegetable broth
>
> 1 cup red lentils, rinsed and drained

Place a stock pot over medium heat. Add the oil, onion, and red pepper. Sauté for 3 minutes, then add the salt, pepper, garlic, coriander, cumin, paprika, and chili powder. Stir to combine, then add the pumpkin, broth, and lentils.

Bring to a boil, then reduce the heat to hold a low simmer. Set the lid on the pot just slightly askew and simmer for 30 minutes. Stir occasionally to make sure nothing is getting stuck to the bottom of the pot.

MICRONUTRIENTS

Micronutrients are vitamins and minerals that the body needs in very small amounts. They are not a direct source of energy but are essential to the body's ability to create energy. The first sign of a nutrient deficiency is fatigue because without appropriate levels of micronutrients, the mitochondria lack what they need to produce energy, or adenosine triphosphate (ATP).

Vitamins can be water soluble, which means the body takes in as much as it needs and excretes the rest. They can also be fat soluble, meaning that they are absorbed and held in the tissues.

Water-Soluble Vitamins

These vitamins cannot be stored in the body, so they need to be replaced daily. Most of the grains, dairy products, fruits, and vegetables we eat contain some water soluble vitamins. They include the B vitamins, which are crucial to helping mitochondria produce energy. The B vitamins are biotin (B_7), folate (B_9), niacin (B_3), pantothenic acid (B_5). riboflavin (B_2), thiamine (B_1), vitamin B_6, and vitamin B_{12}.

The other water-soluble vitamin is vitamin C, also known as ascorbic acid. This vitamin doubles as an antioxidant and supports immune function, cortisol formation, and iron absorption. Ascorbic acid plays an instrumental role in the repair of wounds, especially in injuries to connective tissue, muscles, and ligaments.

Mitochondria

Mitochondria, the energy centers of each cell, are inherited in the womb and have their own DNA. They require thyroid hormones and cortisol to drive the biochemical processes of energy production. They are destroyed by environmental stressors like heavy metals, carbon monoxide, and pesticides as well as internal stress. The body can produce more mitochondria by engaging in movement.

Fat-Soluble Vitamins

They are absorbed through the small intestine and carried through the immune system to the heart before they reach the bloodstream. Eventually they are stored in our tissues. They include vitamins A, D, E, and K.

Vitamin A is an antioxidant crucial for immune, eye, skin, and liver health. Carrots, kale, spinach, and sweet potatoes are high in vitamin A.

Vitamin D_3, or calcitriol, is necessary for immune function, calcium absorption, and cholesterol synthesis. Most bodies can make D_3 when the cholesterol in skin cells absorbs sunlight. Cod, sardines, shrimp, and eggs are good sources of vitamin D_3.

Vitamin E, or alpha tocopherol, is an antioxidant that supports healthy skin cells, protects the skin from UV light, and helps keep blood vessels flexible to maintain balanced blood pressure. Sources of vitamin E include almonds, kiwi, olives, and sunflower seeds.

Vitamin K supports blood clotting and works with vitamin D, calcium, and magnesium to strengthen bones. Vitamin K_1 is absorbed from foods like leafy greens; vitamin K_2 is absorbed by beneficial gut bacteria; vitamin K_3 is the synthetic form.

Minerals

The body needs only small amounts of minerals but can easily become deficient when one or more systems are out of balance. These essential nutrients are divided into two categories: macrominerals and microminerals. The macrominerals are calcium, chloride, magnesium, phosphorus, potassium, and sodium. The microminerals include boron, chromium, copper, iodine, iron, manganese, molybdenum, selenium, silica, vanadium, and zinc. The human body contains only about a teaspoon of microminerals at any given time. They come from healthy water and soil. Interactions between them are common; too much of one will cause a deficiency in another.

Functions of the Macrominerals

Calcium is essential for cellular communication, muscle contraction, blood clotting, and bone density. The thyroid gland helps regulate calcium balance in the body. Food sources include collards, kale, cinnamon, tempeh, and cow's milk.

Chloride combines with hydrogen to form hydrochloric acid (HCl), which helps the stomach break down food. Chloride also helps maintain optimal pH levels in the bloodstream.

Magnesium mimics the actions of the body's "rest and digest" nervous system. It promotes healthy bowel elimination, relaxes blood vessels and smooth muscle tissue, acts as an anti-inflammatory, and is needed for more than 300 enzymatic functions in the body. Leafy greens, legumes, avocados, almonds, and sunflower seeds are good sources of magnesium.

Phosphorus is found in every cell in the body and is part of both DNA and RNA. It performs more functions than any other mineral. It helps maintain cellular immunity. Adenosine triphosphate, ATP, is the body's energy source and is mainly comprised of phosphorous. Because it is so necessary to life, it is prevalent in many foods we eat daily.

Potassium is necessary for cellular enzyme production, nerve conduction, and heart and muscle contraction. It prevents kidney stones, retains calcium to support healthy bones, and helps form the hydrochloric acid that the stomach needs to break down food. Potatoes, winter squash, boy choy, and papaya are high in potassium.

Sodium is essential for nerve conduction and blood pressure regulation. Too much of it depletes calcium and can lead to osteoporosis. Food sources of sodium include winter foods such as liver, beef, seaweed, black beans, and almonds.

Functions of the Microminerals

Boron helps the body convert cholesterol to vitamin D. It is part of boric acid and can be found in almonds, prunes, and raisins.

Chromium enhances the effects of insulin, making it essential for regulating blood glucose. Onions, tomatoes, and romaine lettuce are good sources of it.

Copper is necessary for forming myelin sheathing and melanin. Mitochondria need it to produce ATP. Copper aids in iron absorption but competes with zinc absorption. It is abundant in apricots, cashews, cremini mushrooms, potatoes, quinoa, and sesame seeds.

Iodine supports thyroid function, and deficiency can lead to goiter. Brown rice, eggs, oats, seaweed, strawberries, and turkey are sources of iodine.

Iron is essential for carrying oxygen to mitochondria and for mitochondria to make ATP through the electron transport chain. It enhances immune function and DNA synthesis. Iron is absorbed by the intestines and carried to the bone marrow by transferrin so that red blood cells can be made. Iron is stored as ferritin. Food sources include beef, chlorella (algae), lentils, spinach, turmeric, and venison.

Manganese is necessary for bone development, antioxidant synthesis, and the formation of scar tissue and neurotransmitters. In the brain, manganese activates the process that converts the amino acid glutamate to glutamine, which heals the lining of the digestive tract and feeds colon cells. Food sources include brown rice, chickpeas, flaxseed, oats, pineapple, and spinach.

Molybdenum helps break down proteins and can be found in black beans, milk, and organ meats.

Selenium improves thyroid performance by helping the body convert the inactive form of the thyroid hormone into the active form. The antioxidant glutathione, which soaks up potentially harmful free radicals, needs selenium to be created. Food sources include Brazil nuts, cod, oats, salmon, and tuna.

Silica is essential for healthy skin, nails, and hair, as well as collagen production, the formation of healthy bones and connective tissue, and arterial flexibility. Food sources of silica include beets, bell peppers, brown rice, and oats.

Vanadium works with chromium to balance blood glucose. Corn, parsley, and seafood are rich in this micromineral.

Zinc stimulates the replication of immune cells and activates T lymphocytes. It increases alpha interferon, which stimulates T helper cells to work with B cells to kill off infections. Zinc supports thyroid health, balances blood glucose, and decreases pro-inflammatory cytokines. Beef, lamb, peas, pumpkin seeds, and sesame seeds are good sources of zinc.

FOOD COMBINING FOR HEALTH

Food and mood are deeply interrelated. Depending on what you are noticing in your digestive system, specific supplements, foods, and herbs can be supportive. For example:

- **For diarrhea,** astringent herbs and foods are helpful: amaranth, applesauce, carob, eggs, meadowsweet *(Filipendula ulmaria)*.
- **For constipation,** fibrous foods are supportive: arrowroot, flax-seed meal, pears, sweet potato. Magnesium citrate helps move bowels by promoting smooth muscle contractions.
- **For gassiness and bloating,** bitter foods are essential: artichoke, burdock root, chard, rutabaga, spinach. Digestive bitters are supportive as well: angelica, chamomile, ginger, goldenrod.
- **For sugar cravings and leaky gut,** try supplementing with the amino acid L-glutamine and the probiotic strain *Akkermansia muciniphila,* or eating fatty fish.

Understanding digestive fire, or *agni* in Ayurveda, can help you work toward regaining balance in the gut. Bloating, gassiness, and heartburn can indicate that you have either too little or too much stomach acid. To find out how your digestion functions, you can do the digestive fire test from the Ayurvedic tradition: Drink ½ teaspoon of baking soda in a small glass of warm water after meals. If symptoms improve, you have too much stomach acid, and you should avoid sour, acidic, and spicy foods. If symptoms do not improve with the baking soda, drink 1 tablespoon of apple cider vinegar in a small glass of warm water before meals. If symptoms improve, you have too little stomach acid. Keep drinking apple cider vinegar before meals. Avoid fats and meat and eat cooked beets, celery, and apples as part of your daily meals for a week.

Occasional digestive symptoms such as gas, bloating, or cramping can mean that the body is responding to a food combination that is not ideal. If this is the case for you, know that it is much easier to digest one kind of protein at a time. Mixing beans and meat often makes digestion harder. The body sometimes prefers to digest whole grains and vegetables on their own, without the presence of proteins like meat, dairy, and legumes.

To reset the gut, it may be helpful to eat five smaller meals daily and simplify the kinds of foods eaten during any given meal. This may seem challenging or cumbersome at first, but the body will quickly express its gratitude by reducing many of the symptoms that have been challenging. Consider these simplified combinations:

- Nonstarchy vegetables with protein: broccoli with chicken or nuts; cabbage with eggs; green beans with cheese
- Whole grains, legumes, or starchy vegetables with nonstarchy vegetables: rice, beans, or sweet potato with kale, spinach, or mushrooms
- Fats and oils with nonstarchy vegetables: zucchini with olive oil
- Fruit alone*

Try eating just these simplified food combinations for a week to ten days, and see if any symptoms start to dissipate.

Try to pay attention to the thermal nature of foods as well. If you experience indigestion, eat more cooling foods. If you experience gas and bloating, eat more warming foods. The more we eat in accordance with our ancestry and constitution, the better we feel and the more we learn to appreciate and respect the wisdom of traditional cultures. Return to your discoveries about your constitution. Are you someone who can benefit from more warming foods or more cooling foods? Make a list of foods you enjoy and place them in either the warm, cool, or neutral category.

As we begin to align with the nutrients and energetics we need in a given moment, life begins to feel more joyful and easeful. These foods will change as we change. Intuitive eating and mindfulness create a space for the body to make different requests for nourishment.

---

*According to all traditional nutritional philosophies, raw fruit is best eaten alone. That said, if you always eat a banana and peanut butter for your snack and do not feel any signs of inflammation, please keep doing it. However, if you are notice itchy/puffy eyes, dry throat, achy muscles and/or joints, difficulty falling or staying asleep, itchy skin, gas, bloating, or cramping, you may want to reconsider that snack.

THERMAL PROPERTIES OF FOODS

Food	Cold	Cool	Neutral	Warm	Hot
Vegetables	Cilantro Seaweed Snow peas	Alfalfa sprouts Asparagus Beets Broccoli Cabbage Carrots Cauliflower Celery Corn Cucumbers Lettuce Spinach Summer squash Zucchini	Chard Potatoes Pumpkins Shiitake mushrooms Sweet potatoes Winter squash Yams	Collard greens Green beans Kale Leeks Onions	Garlic Scallions
Fruits	Bananas Grapefruit Pears	Apricots Figs Lemons Oranges Peaches Persimmons Strawberries Tomatoes	Apples Mangos Olives Papayas	Cherries Coconut Dried papaya Grapes Pineapples Plums Raspberries Tangerines	
Grains	Barley Millet Wheat	Brown rice Cornmeal Quinoa Rye	Amaranth Buckwheat Oats Sweet rice		
Seeds and Beans	Chia seeds Pumpkin seeds	Adzuki beans Kidney beans	Almonds Flaxseed Mung beans Pecans	Black beans Lentils Pine nuts Sesame seeds Walnuts	
Animal Products (always hormone- and antibiotic-free)	Pork	Clams Crabs Eggs	Dairy products Fish Oysters	Beef Fish Poultry	Lamb

7

Personalized Nutrition Plans

Nourish Your Body and Spirit

When diet is wrong, medicine is of no use. When diet is correct, medicine is of no need.

AYURVEDIC PROVERB

When I was growing up in Italy, my family's meal plans changed based on the season. Bean soups, hearty stews, and vegetable and rice dishes nourished us in the winter, while asparagus, eggs, homemade egg pasta, and artichokes were spring fare. Fish, fruit, and greens were summer food, while squashes and flatbreads framed autumn meals. When I came to the States, I searched everywhere for that familiar seasonal eating rhythm. It was not in the diners or grocery stores. After traveling to almost all fifty states searching for small, regenerative farms and ancestral foods, I found these food traditions and growing practices in places like Louisiana and New Mexico. These places maintain distinct culinary and cultural heritage. Their inspiration moved me to revive my own.

When I moved to Vermont to become a college student, I found a largely colonized region, yet one that still valued small-scale agriculture: the history of the colonists who overtook indigenous people in this area was based on hunting and diversified farming. I enjoyed planting potatoes at Golden Russet Farm in Shoreham and riding the horses next door. I helped establish college gardens that provide food for campus dining halls today. I lived in the Italian house on campus and was able to cook meals to share with our community of international students.

I had rediscovered my nutritional roots and returned to a whole-foods way of eating. This was not the first time that my eating rhythms would change and then regain balance. Constitution, conditions, and the environment around us all impact our lives. Becoming chronically ill while living in the tropical climate of Indonesia taught me a profound lesson about what it can look like to live in an environment that's not indigenous to an individual's ancestry, genetics, or microbiome. The healing I gained through ayahuasca took place in another tropical environment in Ecuador. After I returned to Vermont post-ayahuasca, I worked diligently to reincorporate foods with the support of mindfulness, intuition, and loved ones.

I could never have successfully healed my gut without supporting my tired and wired nervous system and adrenal glands at the same time. The courage to try new foods, regardless of consequences, came through this support. I learned that I was now lactose and gluten intolerant and felt grounded enough to accept that reality. I came to understand through my studies that refined sugar is a nonfood that is not ideal for anyone to consume, both because of its health implications and because of the negative impact on beet and sugarcane farmers. It took me almost six years to regain the forty pounds I had lost during my twenties and to heal my nervous system. My gut and nerves will forever be more sensitive than they had been. I see this sensitivity as the blessing of illness because it calls me to take care of myself despite my fire-type personality wanting to push boundaries beyond reasonable limits.

Seeing illness as a blessing has allowed me to learn from it and hold space for others to learn as well. The more we take stock of life's transitions and incorporate their teachings as authentic wisdom, the more we can adapt to change with grace. After I regained the weight that parasites had taken from me, I became pregnant. It felt like a magical culmination of so much dedication and a sign of true wellness. With the joy of my first pregnancy came the discovery that my mother's hypothyroidism had been activated in my body, too. I immediately started taking synthetic thyroid hormone to protect my growing baby and changed my way of eating once again to one that centered around protein.

I had an amazing first pregnancy and expected the same when I became pregnant a second time. However, I had another learning experience coming my way: I felt terribly ill for the entirety of the first trimester. I had to let go of my dietary ideals and eat whatever I could keep down to keep myself and my baby alive. Even though it felt horrifying, saltines, almonds, and Gatorade were my life rafts for the first twelve weeks. Our second child is thriving even though I veered so dramatically off my planned dietary path for a period of time. I mention this because I always set out with the best intentions to follow a nutrition plan. However, I am not in control. During that first trimester, I had to embrace the reality before me and trust that it would change.

And change it did. In the thirteenth week of pregnancy, it was as though someone had flipped a switch and I could suddenly eat all the foods that I was accustomed to eating. I know that not all people are so lucky. Many are sick throughout their pregnancy, which is incredibly challenging. Luckily, once babies are born, hormones readjust, and digestion can slowly return to balance. The teaching is that everything changes. Nothing goes back to the way it was before.

When any system goes out of balance and returns to balance, the new version of homeostasis is a new way of being. The poignancy and beauty of this reality are reminders that no part of us is permanent and we have an infinite capacity to rejuvenate ourselves. In fact, transformation is one of our body's main foci. A year into the coronavirus pandemic, just after my second child's first birthday, my health began to take a challenging turn. I had developed the autoimmune version of hypothyroidism, Hashimoto's. I spoke with three different naturopaths, all of whom told me that this was an irreversible condition. In fact, their firm opinions drove me to reverse my condition. It took me a year, but I was able to do it through the support of a new nutrition plan that focused on the immune system. I took eggs, nuts, seeds, legumes, and grains out of my food repertoire for six weeks and then reintroduced them one by one. I learned a lot about what my body could and could not tolerate and came to understand on a deeper level what the immune system needs to reset itself.

When I reported back to the doctors that I had reversed my condition, they reminded me that I could go back into an autoimmune state at any time. I absolutely understand that to be true, yet I do not want to live my life in fear of that happening. While I was working to reverse Hashimoto's, I was bitten by a tick and came down with a raging case of Lyme disease. With the help of a wise friend who is a naturopath, I was able to eradicate the infection from my system over the course of a month. Shortly after reversing my autoimmune condition, the coronavirus came to our house for the first time. I felt thyroid symptoms flare up again and returned to the foods and herbs that healed me. Life is always going to affect how we make decisions about our health. The more we learn through challenge, the better equipped we are to heal ourselves the next time illness arises.

Each of us has unique needs based on our inherent constitution and life journey. By listening to our bodies, we can attune to needs as they change, not only seasonally but also based on circumstances. Please know that the plan you create for yourself now will look different as the seasons change. This awareness is an invitation to constantly tune in to your body with a beginner's mind and be willing to change your plan based on what you notice.

Ideally, this plan goes beyond meals and becomes a nutrition plan that helps you feel fulfilled on all levels. Make a list of foods that feel nourishing and meaningful to you. Perhaps some of them evoke a memory that feeds your soul. Others may be ancestral foods that feel utterly satisfying. For some people, ancestry is complex; if you feel a deeper resonance with one part of your heritage, go toward it in your food choices. There may be less resonant aspects of your family history that you need to unpack and for which you need to make amends in your own life. Take this as an opportunity to embrace what works while still exploring the parts that feel painful so that transformation may occur. Then consider which daily practices support you, beyond the food you eat. For me, those daily rituals include hugs, hikes, herbal tea, stretching, writing, music, and deep breathing.

Keep this list close at hand, especially for those times when you reach for food when you're not hungry or when you feel a sense of self-judgment or sorrow flooding your heart. Let these sources of spiritual nourishment be an island in the sea of your days.

SENSITIVITIES

The only good reason to restrict or eliminate food groups is if you have a sensitivity or allergy to them. The top seven allergens are dairy, eggs, gluten, corn, soy, peanuts, and refined cane sugar. These allergens trigger inflammation for three primary reasons: they contain proteins that are hard to digest, they are highly processed, or they are replete with pesticides and/or antibiotics.

Organically grown heirloom wheat is one of the most nutritious grains available. It has the most balanced profile of protein, fat, and carbohydrate of any grain. No wonder the world loves it. I grew up in Italy eating beautiful homemade pasta and bread made with wheat grown by small-scale farms near my home. However, that's not the case for most people these days. To feed the world's demand for wheat, large-scale agriculture now dominates its production. Commercially produced wheat is treated with pesticides, which lead to food allergies. There has been a dramatic rise in gluten sensitivity both because wheat has been hybridized to maximize yields and because much of the commercially grown wheat on the market is doused with pesticides that disrupt the endocrine (hormonal) system and make the gut dangerously leaky. This means we're eating wheat that our body doesn't recognize because it's been modified and taking in toxins that our body doesn't need because of pesticide residues. Some of us are truly allergic to gluten, as in the case of people with celiac disease and Crohn's disease. Avoiding all glutinous grains is essential for these folks.

For those who are sensitive (not allergic) to gluten and would like to reduce the mucus-forming effects of the gliadin protein that's in wheat, spelt, kamut, einkorn, barley, and rye, first try avoiding it for twenty-one days. Then, one by one and in small amounts, reincorporate glutinous grains, eating only organic, heirloom versions, and see how your system responds.

You can do the same for any food you think you might be sensitive to. First stop eating it for twenty-one days. Then reintroduce it by eating a bit of it at every meal. Notice whether your body, mind, or emotions exhibit any of your trademark inflammatory symptoms. If so, this food may be more challenging for you to digest. This does not mean that you must eliminate this food entirely. It is just a reminder to eat it occasionally as opposed to daily. A true food allergy can trigger severe symptoms like anaphylaxis. If this is the case, you likely already know that you must avoid a certain food as a life-saving measure.

Ingredient Substitutions

Sometimes you can replace inflammatory ingredients with ones that are easier on the body. Here are some ideas (unless otherwise specified the substitution is one to one).

Ingredient: Wheat flour
Substitutes: Spelt flour (wheat-free), half oat flour and half millet flour (gluten-free), half almond flour and half arrowroot flour (grain-free)

Ingredient: Butter
Substitutes: Ghee, coconut oil, half ghee and half olive oil

Ingredient: Eggs
Substitutes: 1 mashed banana or ¼ cup applesauce per egg (best for baked goods), 1 tablespoon agar flakes whisked into

1 tablespoon water and chilled for 5 minutes (for an egg white substitute), 2 tablespoons ground flaxseed mixed with ¼ cup hot water

Ingredient: Cheese sauce or dip
Substitute: 1 cup cashews blended with 1 teaspoon lemon juice and ¼ teaspoon each of nutmeg, salt, and pepper

Ingredient: Oil in baked goods
Substitutes: Applesauce, pureed bananas, pureed cooked prunes

Ingredient: Cooking oil
Substitutes: Vegetable stock, wine, apple cider vinegar

Ingredient: Cream in soup
Substitutes: Hot water whisked with arrowroot flour; apple cider vinegar blended with puréed carrots, onions, and/or garlic; broth whisked with turmeric, cinnamon, and nutmeg; coconut milk

Beet and Cane Sugar Alternatives

Beet and cane sugars are highly processed and ideally avoided because the body must leach minerals from our bones to digest it. Thankfully, there are many alternatives. Below I present a few suggestions. Consider bananas, applesauce, or monk fruit (erythritol-free) as other options.

Coconut sugar: Low on the glycemic index and rich in polyphenols, iron, zinc, calcium, potassium, phosphorus, and other nutrients. It is extracted from the sap of coconut flower blooms, which is heated and then evaporated. Substitute it one to one for cane or beet sugar.

Dates: High in fiber, potassium, copper, iron, manganese, magnesium, and vitamin B_6. From the date palm tree, dates are easily digested and help the body metabolize proteins, fats, and carbohydrates. Chop them and add to your favorite baked goods, or soak them, blend, and substitute for sugar. Use ¼ cup dates for every 1 cup sugar; they are very sweet.

Raw honey: A true superfood, packed with minerals and enzymes that act as natural antibiotics and support the growth of healthy bacteria in the digestive tract. Look for local raw honey.

Maple syrup: Native to North America, it is made by catching the sap from maple trees, evaporating the water, and bottling the resulting syrup. It is minimally processed, prebiotic, probiotic, and packed with minerals such as calcium, manganese, potassium, and zinc. The darker the syrup, the more beneficial nutrients it contains. To use it in baked goods, replace 1 cup sugar with ½ cup maple syrup and add 2 tablespoons extra flour to absorb the extra liquid.

Stevia: Native to South America, it has been used for hundreds of years in that region as a sweetener that supports healthy blood sugar levels. It's easy to grow as an annual in any garden. The dried leaves of one plant will give you over a year's worth of sweetening options. Its constituent steviosides make it more than two hundred times as sweet as sugar. It has no glycemic load or kilocalories. It can lower progesterone levels.

DESIGNING HEALTHY MEALS

Remember that we are all different. Reflect on your constitution. Do you thrive with more protein, more carbohydrates, or a balance of both? Do you prefer to eat your carbohydrates in the evening because they're calming? Does a protein-rich breakfast work best for you? Keep these questions in mind as you create your meal plans and work to identify the guidelines that work best for you.

Here are some suggestions to consider.

- Follow the tenets of the Mediterranean way of eating in constructing a plate: one-third whole grains, one-third vegetables, one-third protein.
- Try to eat a rainbow of fruits and vegetables every day. Produce is loaded with enzymes, vitamins, minerals, fiber, and important

phytonutrients such as carotenoids and bioflavonoids that protect us from illness and help the body detoxify.

- Choose organic and/or local foods whenever possible. At the very least, try to avoid the "Dirty Dozen" (see the box on the following page). Organic and pesticide-free foods have higher levels of nutrients because organic farmers generally pay more attention to their animals' wellness and to the health of the soil.

- Try to eat foods that are in season. Fresh foods are more vital and nourish the organs that align with each time of year.

- Eat foods that will spoil. This ensures that the food still has life in it. Packaged foods lack this nutrient-rich vitality.

- Eat raw fruits alone, at least an hour before or after a meal.

- Eat high-quality fats. The fats found in fatty fish, nuts and seeds, pastured meat, and whole grains provide the essential fatty acids we need to thrive.

- Cook with unrefined vegetable oils, such as sesame, sunflower, or olive oil. When using saturated fats, choose those of the highest quality, such as expeller-pressed organic coconut oil or grass-fed butter.

- Drink pure water. Test your water to learn about its quality. Use a filtering system to remove chlorine and unwanted organic compounds.

- Eat breakfast! This practice jump-starts digestion so you feel more energized, assimilate more nutrients, and use food for energy more effectively.

- When eating a dessert, choose unrefined sweeteners such as honey, maple syrup, or coconut sugar. Avoid cane sugar when possible, as it is highly refined and devoid of the amazing nutrients contained in whole sugar cane.

- Honor all of your food choices with compassion and nonjudgment.

Clean Fifteen and Dirty Dozen

The Environmental Working Group (EWG) has created a shopping guide to help consumers avoid pesticides in produce. The "Dirty Dozen" are those foods that, under conventional agriculture, carry the highest pesticide load, meaning you should buy organic versions or find local varieties grown without pesticides. The "Clean Fifteen" are those foods with the lowest pesticide load, and consequently they are the safest conventionally grown crops to consume from the standpoint of pesticide contamination. As of 2023, these are the EWG lists to consider when shopping and eating produce.

The Clean Fifteen

Asparagus	Onions
Avocados	Papayas
Cabbage	Pineapples
Carrots	Sweet corn
Honeydew melon	Sweet peas (frozen)
Kiwi	Sweet potatoes
Mangos	Watermelons
Mushrooms	

The Dirty Dozen

Apples	Kale, collard, and mustard greens
Bell and hot peppers	Nectarines
Blueberries	Peaches
Cherries	Pears
Grapes	Spinach
Green beans	Strawberries

METABOLISM MYTHS

There are many kinds of bodies in this world. There's a story that some bodies have a fast metabolism, while others have a slow one. This is simply not true. The foods we eat can either accelerate or decelerate metabolism at any given time. Metabolism does increase during the first year of life and decline by 25 percent on average during the last quarter of life. However, throughout the rest of life it remains stable.[1] Body type is more a factor of internal constitution and external conditions than metabolic rate. Herman Pontzer, a professor of evolutionary anthropology, has been working with indigenous populations like the Hadza and the Shuar for decades to understand how metabolism truly functions. His book, *Burn*, explains that all adults have a similar metabolism and can impact it by reducing stress and eating more plant foods.

The term *hormesis* derives from the ancient Greek *hormê,* "to set in motion." The word *hormone* shares this etymology. The concept of hormesis refers to a potentially harmful stimulus that catalyzes a momentary stress response. As philosopher Friedrich Nietzsche famously said, "What doesn't kill me makes me stronger." This concept is reflected in the interrelationship between humans and phytochemicals, or "plant chemicals." Certain plants protect themselves from birds and insects or respond to stressors such as drought by secreting phytochemicals that are slightly toxic. Many of these compounds are bitter in flavor. When we ingest plants with these phytochemicals, such as broccoli or cilantro, the nervous system responds with a short burst of stress, just like the stress that prompted the plants to produce the phytochemicals. This beneficial form of stress prompts the body to detoxify itself.

When we embrace certain activities in small doses, like ending a shower with thirty seconds of cold water or eating plant foods that are subtoxic, our cells respond by rejuvenating themselves. The key concept with hormesis is that a little goes a long way. If I ate five pounds of arugula, I would probably feel ill. If I soaked in a freezing winter stream for more than a few minutes, I might start to develop frostbite. When creating your personal nutrition plan, consider including foods that are subtoxic but beneficial in small quantities.

Plants are epigenetic modulators: they can activate or deactivate certain genes. Phytochemicals such as resveratrol, curcumin, sulfora-phanes, and catechins can help heal the nervous system through phy-tohormesis by placing it under a minimal amount of stress.[2] Grapes, peanuts, cacao, blueberries, and cranberries are rich in resveratrol. Turmeric is high in curcumin. Brassica family vegetables such as broc-coli, kale, collard greens, cabbage, and Brussels sprouts contain sul-foraphanes. Black beans, apricots, strawberries, and cherries contain catechins. When creating your meal plan, focus on the root causes of imbalance in your body that you are trying to balance. Use the sample meal plan below to balance your choices and pick the recipes that resonate with you.

SAMPLE MEAL PLAN: ONE WEEK

Before meals, try to remember to take some deep breaths and give thanks for the nourishment you are about to receive.

The recipes mentioned below can be found in the following pages and the following liquids and snacks can be used throughout the week.

Liquids

In the morning: herbal tea of your choosing, like cinnamon or
    lemon balm tea
Before bed: chamomile-lavender tea or tulsi tea
2 quarts water daily

Snacks

Carrot sticks and Nutty Crackers
Energy Bite or No-Bake Chocolate Cookie

SAMPLE MEAL PLAN: ONE WEEK

	Daily Menu	Cooking and Preparation
Saturday	**Breakfast:** Coconut Blueberry Quinoa **Lunch:** Leftovers from the past week (to finish what you may have in the refrigerator) **Dinner:** Coconut Green Bean Soup with flatbread	**Morning:** Make a double batch of Coconut Blueberry Quinoa. Go food shopping. Pick up necessary ingredients for the week. **Afternoon:** Make Energy Bites and No-Bake Chocolate cookies. **Evening:** Make and serve Coconut Green Bean Soup and a flatbread of your choice; store the leftover soup in the fridge for lunch tomorrow.
Sunday	**Breakfast:** Coconut Blueberry Quinoa **Lunch:** Coconut Green Bean Soup with flatbread **Dinner:** Salmon with broccoli and wild rice	**Afternoon:** Make Cashew Sauce and Artichoke Sauce; store in the fridge. Make Lentil Squash Soup and oven roasted zucchini for dinner tomorrow night; store in the fridge. **Evening:** Make a double batch of salmon, broccoli, and wild rice; store the leftovers in the fridge for lunch tomorrow. Chop the roots for Tuesday's Healing Bowl dinner; store them raw in the fridge.
Monday	**Breakfast:** Breakfast Muffins **Lunch:** Salmon with broccoli and wild rice **Dinner:** Lentil Squash Soup with oven roasted zucchini and flatbread	**Morning:** Make a double batch of Breakfast Muffins—one for today, one for tomorrow. Pack a lunch if you are going out. **Evening:** Heat and serve the soup and zucchini with flatbread (made earlier in the week).
Tuesday	**Breakfast:** Breakfast Muffins **Lunch:** Lentil Squash Soup with oven roasted zucchini and flatbread **Dinner:** Healing Bowl	**Morning:** Pack a lunch if you are going out. **Evening:** Roast 2 pounds of chicken legs (which should be enough for dinner tonight, lunch tomorrow, and the Greek-Style Lemon Fennel Soup you'll have later in the week). At the same time, roast the roots you chopped the night before. Cook quinoa and greens and combine them with the roasted roots to make the Healing Bowl. Make the Egg Muffins.

SAMPLE MEAL PLAN: ONE WEEK (CONT.)

	Daily Menu	Cooking and Preparation
Wednesday	**Breakfast:** Egg Muffins **Lunch:** Roasted Chicken with Roasted Roots and Cashew Sauce **Dinner:** Frittata with quinoa and Artichoke Sauce	**Morning:** Pack a lunch if you are going out. **Evening:** Prepare the frittata and quinoa; serve with Artichoke Sauce.
Thursday	**Breakfast:** Egg Muffins **Lunch:** Frittata with quinoa **Dinner:** Greek-Style Lemon Fennel Soup	**Morning:** Pack a lunch if you are going out. **Evening:** Prepare Greek-Style Lemon Fennel Soup; store leftovers in the fridge for lunch tomorrow.
Friday	**Breakfast:** Sweet Potato Breakfast Bars with almond butter **Lunch:** Greek-Style Lemon Fennel Soup **Dinner:** Leftovers!	**Morning:** Make sweet potato breakfast bars; pack a lunch if you are going out. **Evening:** Enjoy leftovers from the past week.

Shopping List

Unless a quantity is specified, choose the amount of any item that feels supportive to you.

Fresh Produce

Apples

Avocados—2

Beets

Broccoli

Carrots—5 pounds

Celery

Delicata squash—4 medium

Fennel—1 bulb

Garlic—3 heads

Ginger—1 good-size root

Green beans—1 pound

Kale—3 bunches

Lemons—2

Onions

Rutabagas

Spinach—10 ounces

Sweet potatoes—6 medium

Zucchini—5 or 6 medium

Refrigerated and Frozen Goods

Eggs—2 dozen (or more if you like hard-boiled eggs as a snack)

Plant-based milk

Chicken legs/thighs—2 pounds

Salmon—1 pound

Sauerkraut

Coconut yogurt (unsweetened)

Frozen blueberries

Pantry Goods

Coconut oil

Olive oil

Apple cider vinegar

Whole-grain mustard

Almond butter

Sunflower seed butter
   (organic, no sugar added)

Tahini

Coconut milk

Applesauce (unsweetened)

Artichoke hearts—glass jar

Bulk Goods

Kombu

Oats (quick-cooking)

Quinoa

Red lentils

Wild rice

Almond flour

Arrowroot flour

Coconut flour

Chia seeds

Pumpkin seeds

Almonds

Cashews

Walnuts

Dates

Shredded coconut
   (unsweetened)

Baking powder

Baking soda

Cocoa powder (unsweetened)

Allspice

Cayenne

Cinnamon

Cloves

Coriander

Cumin

Curry powder

Ginger

Nutmeg

Oregano

Paprika

Thyme

Turmeric

Unrefined sea salt

Fresh cracked black pepper

Maple syrup

Raw honey

RECIPES FOR MEAL PLAN

What follows are recipes included in the sample meal plan. Get creative and adapt them to fit your personal tastes, nourishment needs, and meal plan. Here we have categorized them by traditional meal type (breakfast, lunch, dinner, snack) but you can of course eat them any time of day that works for you!

BREAKFAST RECIPES

☙ Breakfast Muffins

> ½ cup arrowroot flour
>
> I cup almond flour*
>
> ¼ cup coconut flour
>
> I teaspoon ground cinnamon
>
> ¼ teaspoon ground nutmeg
>
> ¼ teaspoon ground ginger
>
> I teaspoon baking soda
>
> ½ teaspoon baking powder
>
> ½ teaspoon salt
>
> I tablespoon apple cider vinegar
>
> I cup grated carrots
>
> I cup chopped walnuts
>
> ½ cup cashew or coconut yogurt
>
> ¼ cup olive oil, plus a bit for oiling the muffin pan, if needed
>
> 3 eggs or I cup unsweetened applesauce

Preheat the oven to 350°F. Oil the cups of a muffin pan with olive oil or line them with paper liners.

Combine the flours, spices, baking soda, baking powder and salt in a large bowl. Whisk until blended.

Add the carrots and walnuts to the bowl. Stir together just until the flour mixture is evenly moistened.

---

*Note: You can replace the almond flour with a 1:1 mixture of ground pumpkin seeds and ground sunflower seeds. Grind each seed separately in an espresso bean grinder.

In a separate bowl, whisk together the oil, vinegar, yogurt and eggs or applesauce. Add to the flour mixture and stir just until combined. Spoon the batter into the muffin pan.

Bake for 30 minutes, or until the tops are golden brown and a toothpick inserted into the center comes out clean.

🍉 Coconut Blueberry Quinoa

1½ cups quinoa

2 cups full-fat, organic coconut milk

1 cup water

1 teaspoon vanilla extract

¼ teaspoon salt

¼ teaspoon ground cardamom

¼ teaspoon ground cinnamon

½ cup fresh or frozen blueberries

¼ cup chia seeds

Combine the quinoa, coconut milk, water, vanilla, salt, cardamom, and cinnamon in a small saucepan. Bring to a boil, then reduce the heat and simmer, covered, for 15 minutes. There should still be a bit of liquid left in the pot.

Add the blueberries and chia seeds, mix well, and serve.

🍉 Egg Muffins

2 tablespoons Greek-style or plant-based yogurt

12 eggs

¼ cup dairy-free pesto

½ teaspoon salt

½ teaspoon freshly ground black pepper

Preheat the oven to 350°F. Oil the cups of a muffin pan with olive oil or line them with paper liners.

Whisk all the ingredients together in a mixing bowl.

Fill 12 muffin cups and bake for 18 to 20 minutes.

❦ Sweet Potato Breakfast Bars

For the crust:

>   1 cup quinoa
>   1 cup almond flour
>   ½ cup walnuts
>   ½ teaspoon ground cinnamon
>   ¼ teaspoon ground cardamom
>   A pinch of salt
>   2 tablespoons olive oil, plus a bit for oiling the baking dish
>   1 tablespoon maple syrup
>   1 egg, beaten, or ¼ cup flaxseed meal

For the topping:

>   1 pound sweet potatoes
>   ¼ cup plant milk
>   2 eggs, beaten (optional; omit for a vegan version)
>   2 tablespoons flaxseed meal
>   2 tablespoons maple syrup
>   ½ teaspoon vanilla extract
>   ½ teaspoon ground cinnamon
>   ¼ teaspoon ground ginger
>   ¼ teaspoon ground nutmeg
>   ⅛ teaspoon ground allspice

Start with the sweet potatoes for the topping: Chop and boil the sweet potatoes. Leave the skin on for maximum nutritional benefit. Drain them and set aside.

Meanwhile, make the crust: Cook the quinoa in 2 cups of water.

Preheat the oven to 375°F. Oil an 8 x 8-inch baking dish with olive oil.

Place all crust ingredients in a food processor bowl and pulse until mixture reaches a coarse meal that's evenly moist.

Transfer the mixture to the prepared pan and press it evenly into the bottom. Bake the crust for 15 minutes. Remove from the oven.

Place all the topping ingredients in the food processor and blend until smooth. (There's no need to wash the processor between the crust and the topping.) Pour the mixture onto the crust and smooth the top evenly with a spatula.

Bake for about 25 minutes.

Allow to cool for completely before slicing. Store in the fridge and reheat in an oven or toaster oven.

LUNCH AND DINNER RECIPES

✌ Coconut Green Bean Soup

> 2 tablespoons coconut oil
> 1 onion, diced
> 2 cloves garlic, crushed
> 2 stalks celery, chopped
> 1 rutabaga or 3 parsnips, sliced
> 2 carrots, sliced
> 1 pound green beans, trimmed
> 1 teaspoon salt
> 1 teaspoon freshly ground black pepper
> 1 teaspoon ground coriander
> 1 teaspoon ground cumin
> 1 teaspoon dried thyme
> ¼ teaspoon ground nutmeg
> 4 cups chicken or vegetable stock
> 1 cup coconut milk

Melt the oil in a medium saucepan over medium heat. Add the onion, garlic, celery, carrots, and rutabaga or parsnips. Cook, stirring occasionally, until softened, about 10 minutes. Add the green beans, salt, pepper, coriander, cumin, thyme, and nutmeg. Cook for 5 to 10 minutes more.

Pour in the stock and bring to a boil, then reduce the heat and simmer, covered, for 30 minutes or until the beans are cooked through.

Stir in the coconut milk.

Remove the soup from the heat. Puree in a food processor or blender or with an immersion blender until the consistency is to your liking.

Greek-Style Lemon Fennel Soup

> 2 quarts chicken or vegetable stock
> ½ cup quinoa
> 1 bulb fennel, thinly sliced
> 1 head garlic, cloves separated, peeled, and chopped
> 1-inch piece of kombu seaweed, chopped
> 1 teaspoon ground coriander
> 1 teaspoon ground cumin
> 1 teaspoon freshly ground black pepper
> 1 teaspoon salt
> ½ teaspoon ground cayenne pepper
> ½ cup fresh lemon juice
> ½ cup cashew or coconut yogurt (unsweetened)
> 2 cups shredded chicken or white beans
> ¼ cup chopped fresh fennel fronds

Pour the stock into a soup pot. Add the quinoa, fennel, garlic, kombu, coriander, cumin, pepper, salt, and cayenne. Bring to a boil. Cover, reduce the heat to medium-low, and simmer for 15 minutes, or until the quinoa is cooked. Remove the pot from the heat.

Whisk together the lemon juice and yogurt.

Add the shredded chicken or beans and fennel fronds to the soup. Add the lemon-yogurt mixture, stir, and serve immediately.

Lentil Squash Soup

> 1 cup red lentils, rinsed well
> 2 tablespoons olive oil
> 1 yellow onion, diced
> Salt

2 carrots, diced

2 stalks celery, diced

I medium delicata squash, peeled, seeded, and cut into
½-inch cubes

I teaspoon ground coriander

I teaspoon ground cumin

½ teaspoon ground cinnamon

½ teaspoon ground turmeric

5 cups chicken or vegetable broth

I inch chopped kombu seaweed

I cup chopped kale

I-inch piece of kombu or wakame seaweed, chopped

Soak the lentils in water for 30 minutes. Drain the water, rinse the lentils, and place them in a stock pot with 4 cups water. Do not add salt—this causes flatulence and stomach pain. Simmer for 20 minutes, or until the lentils are soft. Drain off any excess water and set aside.

Heat the olive oil in a soup pot over medium heat. Add the onion and a pinch of salt and sauté until translucent, about 5 minutes.

Add the carrots, celery, delicata squash, and another pinch of salt and sauté until all of the vegetables are just tender, about 5 minutes.

Add the spices and lentils and stir to coat.

Pour in ½ cup of the broth to deglaze the pot, stirring to loosen any bits stuck to the bottom, and cook until the liquid is reduced by half.

Add the remaining 4½ cups broth. Bring to a boil, then reduce the heat to low and add the kale. Cover and simmer for 15 minutes.

☜ Healing Bowl

       Cooked quinoa

       Roasted roots (see below)

       Cooked chicken or beans

       Braised kale

       Lacto-fermented vegetables, as desired

       Sauce of choice

To cook the quinoa: Simmer ½ cup quinoa in 2 cups chicken broth. Add a pinch of salt as the quinoa cooks.

To braise the kale: Fill a large shallow saucepan or medium pot with ½ inch of water. Chop 1 bunch of kale. Place the chopped kale in the pot. Sprinkle with salt. Cover the pot and turn the heat up to high. Once the water begins to boil, turn the heat down to low and braise for about 5 minutes, or until all the water is gone.

For sauces: Try Cashew Sauce (page 178), Artichoke Sauce (page 178), Macadamia Nut Sauce (page 139), or your favorite homemade blend of fresh herbs, lemon, olive oil, and salt.

For the lacto-fermented vegetables: Try fermented carrots (page 112), kimchi (page 111), or sauerkraut.

To assemble: Place the quinoa, roasted root vegetables, and chicken or beans in a bowl. Add a generous serving of greens. Top with a forkful of lacto-fermented veggies. Spoon a sauce over the top and enjoy!

☜ Roasted Roots

Feel free to substitute any root vegetables you prefer. Adapting recipes to suit your own tastes and needs is important!

       3 medium beets

       1 sweet potato

       2 carrots

       1 rutabaga or 2 parsnips

       ¼ cup olive oil

       Salt and freshly ground black pepper

Preheat the oven to 400°F.

Wash all the vegetables. Chop into bite-sized pieces. Place on a baking sheet or in a glass baking dish. Toss everything with olive oil, salt, and pepper.

Roast for 45 minutes, or until the beets are fork tender. Remove from the oven and enjoy.

🍉 Roasted Chicken

> Chicken legs and thighs, bone-in
> Salt and freshly ground black pepper

Preheat the oven to 400°F.

Put the chicken in a glass baking dish. Sprinkle with salt and pepper. Bake for 45 minutes. Remove from the oven and enjoy.

🍉 Frittata

> 3 tablespoons olive oil, plus a bit for oiling the pie plate
> ½ yellow onion, thinly sliced
> ¼ teaspoon salt
> 1 carrot, shredded
> 1 cup fresh spinach
> 8 eggs

Preheat the oven to 400°. Oil a 9-inch pie plate with olive oil.

Heat the oil in a skillet over medium heat. Add the onion and sauté until tender and golden, about 7 minutes. Add the carrot and sauté for another 5 minutes. Add the spinach and cook for another minute, until just wilted.

Transfer the sautéed veggies to the pie plate.

Crack the eggs into a large bowl, add the salt, and beat well with a fork. Pour the beaten eggs into the pie plate and use the fork to press the vegetables down into the egg mixture so that the eggs cover the veggies completely.

Place in the oven and bake until the top is set and lightly golden, about 25 minutes. Cut into wedges and enjoy.

❧ Rosemary-Thyme Flatbread

2 cups almond flour

¼ cup coconut flour

¼ cup flaxseed meal

I teaspoon salt

I teaspoon baking powder

I teaspoon baking soda

I tablespoon dried rosemary

I tablespoon dried thyme

I egg, beaten, or ¼ cup unsweetened applesauce

¼ cup olive oil, plus a bit for oiling the baking sheet

¼ cup plant milk

Preheat the oven to 350°F. Oil a baking sheet with olive oil.

Mix all the ingredients together in the order listed. Spread the mixture in a thin, even layer on the baking sheet.

Bake for 35 minutes, then broil on high for I to 2 minutes to get the top crispy. Enjoy!

❧ Shredded Vegetable Flatbread

I cup almond flour

½ cup arrowroot flour

3 tablespoons flaxseed meal

½ teaspoon dried thyme

¼ teaspoon salt

¼ teaspoon ground nutmeg

I cup shredded carrots

½ cup shredded zucchini

3 tablespoons olive oil, plus a bit for oiling the baking dish

¼ cup plant milk

I egg, beaten, or ¼ cup unsweetened applesauce

Preheat the oven to 350°F. Oil a glass baking dish.

Mix all the ingredients together in the order listed. Press the mixture into oiled baking dish.

Bake for 35 minutes.

☺ Focaccia Flatbread

> 1 cup almond flour
>
> ½ cup arrowroot flour
>
> ¼ cup coconut flour
>
> 3 tablespoons flaxseed meal
>
> 2 tablespoons hemp seeds
>
> 1 teaspoon sea salt
>
> ½ teaspoon baking soda
>
> ¼ cup plant milk (unsweetened)
>
> ¼ cup olive oil, plus a bit for oiling the baking dish
>
> 2 eggs, beaten, or ¼ cup unsweetened applesauce
>
> 2 tablespoons chopped fresh chives, rosemary, and/or thyme
>
> 2 cloves garlic, chopped
>
> Flaky sea salt or kosher salt, for sprinkling on top

Preheat the oven to 400°F. Oil an 8 x 8-inch baking dish with olive oil.

Combine the flours, flaxseed, hemp seeds, salt, and baking soda in a large bowl. Whisk together.

Make a well in the center and add the remaining ingredients. Mix these ingredients with each other and then incorporate the dry mixture into the wet one, mixing well.

Pour the batter into prepared dish and level with a spatula. Sprinkle with flaked salt and bake for 15 minutes.

Let cool for at least 10 minutes before slicing.

SAUCE RECIPES

☙ Cashew Sauce

> I cup raw cashews, soaked in hot water for 30 minutes
> or in cool water overnight
> I cup unsweetened almond milk
> 2 teaspoons lemon juice
> I¼ teaspoons apple cider vinegar
> ½ teaspoon maple syrup
> ¼ teaspoon sea salt, or to taste
> I pinch freshly ground black pepper

Place all the ingredients in a food processor and blend well.
Enjoy! Store in the fridge, where the sauce will keep for up to
I week.

☙ Artichoke Sauce

> I (8-ounce) jar artichoke hearts in water
> ¼ cup olive oil
> ½ tablespoon fresh lemon juice
> ½ tablespoon dried thyme
> ½ teaspoon sea salt

Drain the artichokes, then put them in a blender with the
remaining ingredients. Blend at the highest speed for 2 minutes.
Enjoy! This sauce is especially good with baked chicken and
zucchini, crackers, or quinoa and roasted root veggies. Store in
the fridge, where the sauce will keep for up to 2 weeks.

SNACK RECIPES

☙ Nutty Crackers

        1 cup pumpkin seeds

        1 cup sunflower seeds

        1 cup almond flour

        ½ cup arrowroot flour

        3 tablespoons flaxseed meal

        ½ teaspoon salt

        ½ teaspoon ground coriander

        ½ teaspoon dried thyme

        ¼ cup olive oil

        ½ cup boiling water

Preheat the oven to 300°F. Line a baking sheet with parchment paper.

Combine the pumpkin seeds, sunflower seeds, almond flour, and arrowroot flour in a bowl and mix well.

Add the flaxseed, salt, coriander, thyme, olive oil, and boiling water and mix well, until a thick dough forms. If mixture seems a bit dry, add a few more splashes of water.

Spread the mixture in a thin layer on the parchment-lined baking sheet.

Bake for 45 minutes. Then turn off the oven and let the cracker tray sit in the oven to cool and crisp up for an hour or so.

Let cool completely before breaking into cracker pieces. Store at room temperature in paper bags.

☻ Energy Bites

    1 cup almond butter

    2 tablespoons maple syrup or raw honey*

    1 cup unsweetened shredded coconut

    ⅓ cup flaxseed meal

    ⅓ cup coarsely chopped pumpkin seeds

    1 teaspoon chia seeds

    ½ teaspoon ground cinnamon

    A pinch of salt

Mix the almond butter and maple syrup or honey until smooth.

Add all the other ingredients and mix well.

Mix in more coconut as needed to make dough thick.

Roll the dough into small balls. You can also spread the mixture on a baking sheet and cut into squares.

Store the balls in an airtight container in a cool place. They will keep for 1 week.

---

*If you prefer to have no glycemic load, use monk fruit extract in place of the maple syrup or honey. I prefer the liquid version. It only takes about 6 drops to make a dish like Energy Bites extremely sweet.

☻ No-Bake Chocolate Cookies

    1 cup unsweetened shredded coconut

    ¼ cup chopped pecans

    ⅓ cup almond butter

    ¼ cup unsweetened cacao powder

    ¼ cup coconut oil

    3 tablespoons maple syrup*

    ½ teaspoon vanilla extract

    ½ teaspoon ground cinnamon

---

*If you prefer to have no glycemic load, use monk fruit extract (5 drops) in place of the maple syrup.

Mix all the ingredients together and shape into balls with your hands. Place in a glass container and freeze for 30 minutes or refrigerate for 2 hours.

MEAL PLANNING BY CATEGORY

Here's another way to look at meal planning: Plan a category of dinner for each night of the week, and improvise ingredients within that rotating plan.

Saturdays: Tacos (for example, corn tortillas, beans, roasted sweet potatoes, avocado, salsa, salad greens/sautéed kale)

Sundays: Pasta (for example, pasta with grilled/baked chicken or tempeh, artichoke hearts, olives, spinach, and garlic)

Mondays: Soup (for example, chicken broth with leftover grilled chicken, roasted sweet potatoes, kale, pressed garlic)

Tuesdays: Stir fry (for example, onions, ginger, carrots, bok choy, garlic, mushrooms, tamari and adzuki beans over brown rice)

Wednesdays: Breakfast for dinner (for example, scrambled eggs with Cashew Sauce, mushrooms, and peppers, served with flatbread topped with pesto)

Thursdays: Casserole (for example, leftover stir fry baked with cornmeal, eggs, and yogurt into a quiche, served with salad or steamed broccoli)

Fridays: Leftovers day (enjoy leftovers from the week's meals)

ADAPTING RECIPES

Cookbooks can make it seem that a written recipe is a set of codified rules that should not be broken. But for me, most of the "recipes" I use today were passed down to me orally from my dad and grandmother. They are part of our family's oral tradition. When we start to tell the story of a recipe, where we first learned it, and how we may have adapted it over the years, we are also aware that the nature of life is change. The base story of the recipe is the same (onions, carrots, celery, stock, and rice), but the finishing touches are different.

The more we get creative with basic recipes and adapt them to what's happening in the moment or what produce is available seasonally, the more we align with ourselves and our environment. As an example, I had always made pizza dough with wheat flour, water, salt, yeast, and olive oil, the way my dad taught me. When I was chronically ill, I couldn't digest wheat flour, and I missed my dad's pizza. Eventually I tried making pizza with a cauliflower crust. The scent coming from the oven as it baked brought me to tears remembering Friday nights in our apartment growing up. The pizza was delicious and I was actually able to savor it.

Indeed, the sense of taste is olfactory. We taste first with our noses. This is the reason why I encourage people to smell their food before they eat it. Not only does this practice awaken the salivary glands and prepare the pancreas to secrete the digestive enzymes needed to process our food, but it also awakens the pleasure centers in our brain that prime us to enjoy the experience of eating. I have been cooking every day for as long as I can remember, first with my father and my grandmother, then with anyone who would join me. For me, the "joy of cooking" comes both from preparing the food itself and from anticipating the opportunity to sit down and savor it.

Mastering the art of cooking, as Julia Child might say, is about finding your joy. What sparks passion for you? In the end, we can eat food prepared with love using whole, local, pesticide-free ingredients. We can be mindful of how we eat and take action to intervene in a corporate food system that takes the power away from its consumers. However, I know now that the path to longevity and vitality is enjoying this moment. Whether we're eating saltines or boeuf bourguignon, we are eating food, which sustains us and allows us to spend another precious day on this Earth.

I trust that I have brought inspiration and joy to others who have tried recipes that I have shared and pondered the role of food in their own lives. I always encourage you to adapt any recipe to your needs and palate. The beauty of preparing food is our ability to get lost in the process.

8

Simplify

Eating for a Reset

Season food with the proper amount of salt at the proper moment; choose the optimal medium of fat to convey the flavor of your ingredients; balance and animate those ingredients with acid; apply the right type and quantity of heat for the proper amount of time—do all this and you will turn out vibrant and beautiful food, with or without a recipe.

SAMIN NOSRAT

Periodically simplifying what and how we eat can be a radical act of trusting the body. But it's also an important one, because it allows us to get to the root cause of health issues, which is fundamental to reversing disease and restoring balance.

If the body isn't properly assimilating nutrients and eliminating waste, it's much harder to feel well. Addressing digestion, assimilation, and elimination by simplifying our eating goes a long way in expediting the healing process.

Organs to Address

When we simplify our eating as part of a plan to reset our system, we can target the organs that are primarily involved in digestion and detoxification. The liver and gallbladder, for example, are crucial to healthy digestion. They produce, store, and release bile to break down food in the stomach. The liver and gallbladder need specific nutrients to function properly; otherwise, toxins are not eliminated but released into the bloodstream. In addition to the liver, the kidneys and bladder filter toxins from the blood and return minerals to the bloodstream to maintain electrolyte balance and stable blood pressure.

HELP THE BODY MOVE TOXINS

Our relationship to sugar often has to do with how we were raised. Think back to the role that sweet treats and desserts played in your childhood. Did you receive them as a reward? Were they forbidden? Did desserts flow freely daily? These patterns get set up at an early age and become ingrained.

Food is emotional. Whether or not we're eating because of hunger, stress, boredom, self-judgment, or compulsion, food can help either calm us down or rev us up. By redefining the way we relate to food and eating, we can shift our emotional center back to what's really going on for us. We can step out of our conditioning and our stress response and live in the moment with food.

Sugar is highly addictive, and overconsumption generates chronic stress symptoms in the body. Why? Because our bodies can't keep up with the amount of insulin and glycogen needed to metabolize foods high in processed sugars.

At the same time, when the body is under stress, it seeks sub-stances to calm that stress—including sugar. Although soothing momentarily, especially if we are feeling emotional or exhausted, it sends our bodies on a blood sugar roller coaster that leaves us want-ing more. The body eventually starts to operate in chronic survival mode, releasing far more stress hormones (cortisol, epinephrine, and norepinephrine) than we need into the bloodstream. Chronic stress leads to inflammation, decreased immunity, insomnia, weight gain, and insulin resistance.

During a time of nutritional simplification, the body will get off the roller coaster and be able to enjoy sweetness in a more bal-anced way. As the body eliminates toxins that naturally build up over time, there is an improvement in symptoms of imbalances. Lack of energy or fibromyalgia will shift into more sustained energy through-out the day. Brain fog, anxiety, and depression will transform into a more calm and present mental state. Rashes and other skin condi-tions will dissipate. Pain in the joints and muscles and headaches will lessen. Digestive function will become more regular as blood glucose becomes more balanced.

When a particular imbalance has become chronic, the body believes that the imbalance reflects homeostasis, even though this is not the case. Seasonal dietary simplification can help the body reset to a true place of balance and even prevent the development of more serious conditions like autoimmune disorders and cancer. Because the immune system gains support when it doesn't have to deal with inflammatory foods, it can function more effectively instead of being taxed by oxidative stress.

As the immune system restores itself, the nervous system also can heal frayed nerve endings and restore communication between the various branches of the nervous system and the endocrine system, also known as the glands. When inflammation is reduced in both the immune and nervous systems, other organs function more effec-tively. However, imbalance comes not only from what we put into our bodies, but also from what we are exposed to in our environment.

Environmental toxins include not only pesticides in foods, but also plastics, packaging materials, furnishings, and chemicals used to treat lawns and make household cleaning products and body care products. Certain homes or workplaces can be prone to developing mold or have chemicals in their water pipes or walls.

The body can detoxify these chemicals and pesticides for some period of time but eventually becomes too taxed to properly eliminate them from the system. Supporting the detoxification process through seasonal nutritional simplification is an age-old way of healing. In ancestral cultures, this process happened naturally because of seasonal food availability or lack thereof.

Recognizing Chronic Inflammation

When we have been feeling "off" or out of balance for three months or longer, it's likely that some system in our body is imbalanced, and because all systems in the body are interrelated, the effects spread and trigger other symptoms. Many of the foods we eat regularly, even the ones that are considered "healthy," may at certain times challenge digestion. Simplifying by eating seasonally gives the body an opportunity to speak with us and creates space for us to hear its messages.

Signs of Inflammation

Lymphatic: puffy eyes, dark circles around the eyes, fatigue

Nervous system: difficulty staying asleep, occasional anxiety or depression, confusion, headache

Gastrointestinal: drowsiness after meals, gas, bloating, nausea, belching, constipation, diarrhea

Musculoskeletal: joint pain, stiffness, swelling, heart palpitations

Respiratory: scratchy throat, itchy ears, shortness of breath, runny nose, chest congestion

Skin: rash, edema, eczema

ONE-DAY BONE BROTH FAST

Some people periodically give their digestive system a rest by fasting for a day. This kind of fast helps shift any eating habits that are no longer working and encourages present moment awareness. I suggest drinking bone broth during a fasting day. When I was growing up, we would often start our evening meal in the colder months with a warm cup of broth. This was the same broth my father made each week to serve as the foundation of our minestrone, goulash, risotto, and other dishes. We would savor a cup of broth and enjoy eating *bollito,* the boiled vegetables and chicken from the broth pot. The creamy, spicy-sweet flavor of the broth-boiled onions was always my favorite.

I have carried the habit of drinking broth into my life as a tool to reset. The broth itself, with its collagen content, is healing for the gut. A periodic bone broth day can reduce inflammation and promote autophagy, the cleanup of dead cells. I suggest drinking up to a gallon of broth, depending on hunger levels. It's wonderful to also drink water and herbal tea alongside the broth. For those who do not feel satiated by just broth, adding a piece of salmon or chicken poached in broth can feel supportive in the middle of the day.

TEN-DAY SIMPLIFIED NUTRITION PLAN

Simplifying your nutritional intake for ten days is a supportive way to detoxify, support digestion, reduce inflammation, and reset your whole system. I like to do it twice a year, usually in April and November, though you can do it anytime you like. It's a great way to jump-start the body's own internal healing capacity.

Foods to Avoid
Here are some foods to avoid when simplifying your eating.

Most grains: barley, einkorn, kamut, oats, rice, spelt, wheat
Corn

Soy products: miso, soy milk, tamari, tempeh, tofu

Beans (though lentils are acceptable)

Dairy products, whether cow, goat, or sheep

Beef and pork

Sweeteners: agave nectar, beet/cane sugar, honey, maple syrup, and all others

Alcohol

Most fruit, including dried fruit

Nightshade family of vegetables: eggplant, peppers, potatoes, tomatoes

Most caffeine: one cup of green tea daily is okay

Refined/processed foods: bread, chips, cookies, crackers, pasta, popcorn, tortillas, and so on

Certain oils: canola, corn, peanut, soy

Foods to Enjoy

The following foods are easy to digest, nutritive, and anti-inflammatory—they tend to work well as a system reset. As always, listen to your body and honor that some of these foods might not resonate with you.

Gluten-free grains: Enjoy amaranth, buckwheat groats, kasha (toasted buckwheat groats), millet (avoid if you have thyroid issues), and quinoa. These anti-inflammatory grains contain many essential amino acids that support the body's rejuvenation process.

Nourishing oils: Use avocado oil, coconut oil, flaxseed oil (do not cook; use only as a garnish), grapeseed oil, olive oil. These oils are anti-inflammatory and promote effective digestion of carbohydrates.

Nuts and seeds: Enjoy pecans, pumpkin seeds, sesame seeds, sunflower seeds, and walnuts. (Though if you believe you have an auto-immune condition, avoid all nuts and seeds.) Otherwise, enjoy between two tablespoons and ¼ cup daily. Avoid nut butters, though, for the duration of the simplified way of eating, as they can lead to mucus in the intestines.

All vegetables except those in the nightshade family: Dandelion greens, dark leafy greens, horseradish, and turnips help detoxify the liver and cleanse the intestines. Try to cook most vegetables; a salad of raw greens up to three times weekly is okay. Include daikon radish and burdock root in your sautés; they support lymphatic detoxification.

Fruit: Enjoy avocados and blueberries. But note that avocados have fermentable oligosaccharides, which could make them hard to digest. If you wonder whether you are sensitive to avocados, please avoid them and then reintroduce them.

Seaweed: Add kelp or kombu to steams, sautés, and soups. Sprinkle dulse flakes on food before you eat it. Seaweed detoxifies the lymphatic system, stabilizes stress hormones, and supports balanced blood glucose.

Animal foods: Pastured/organic poultry and eggs, broth, herring, sardines, and wild-caught salmon are great choices. Consider adding collagen powder (I like the Ancient Nutrition brand) to warm water to create a healing broth.

Lentils: If you are looking for vegetarian protein, eat lentils but avoid beans. Lentils are much easier to digest.

Spices: Focus on cilantro, cinnamon, coriander, cumin, fenugreek, garlic, ginger, thyme, and turmeric to support the reset. These spices are detoxifying, anti-inflammatory, and strengthening to the digestive system.

Fermented foods: Try to eat two tablespoons of sauerkraut, kimchi, or some other lacto-fermented vegetables daily (if you tolerate them and do not have a yeast overgrowth condition). Enjoy ¼ cup of unsweetened coconut or cashew yogurt daily as a snack. If you notice bloating or gassiness after eating fermented foods, it may be time to explore whether you have dysbiosis, or bacterial imbalance, in your gut.

Spice Blends

Try these spice blends to change the flavor palate of simple grains, vegetables, or proteins. Any of them would be appropriate to use for a simplified eating plan.

Bedouin style: black pepper, caraway seeds, cardamom, turmeric, and salt

Central American style: black pepper, cayenne, cumin, oregano, and paprika, with minced fresh garlic and onion

Lebanese style: sesame seeds, sumac, thyme, and salt, all toasted with olive oil and then ground in a mortar and pestle

Mediterranean style: basil, oregano, rosemary, and thyme with minced fresh garlic

North Asian style: coriander, fennel seed, garam masala, cumin, and turmeric with minced fresh garlic and ginger

Sicilian style: black pepper, orange zest, thyme, chopped hazelnuts, and salt

To make a marinade for meat, tempeh, zucchini, or other vegetables, mix any one of these spice blends with equal parts olive oil, vinegar, and water.

Simple Eating Suggestions

- **Make eating a sacred ritual.** Begin meals with a prayer or an expression of gratitude or by simply taking three to five slow breaths with your eyes closed. This prepares the body to receive the food.
- **Eat in a calm environment** where there is little to no distraction. Turn off the television, electronic devices, and music. Avoid excessive conversation, and steer away from conversations about emotionally intense issues.

- **Chew your food until it is of an even consistency.** This requires your attention to be on the food in your mouth. Chewing properly improves digestion and the absorption of the food.
- **Eat at a moderate pace and until you are only about three-quarters full.** Overeating is one of the major causes of disease in our society. When you eat too much, digestion becomes difficult. When you finish eating, you should not feel heavy but you should also not feel hungry. You want to feel satisfied.
- **Drink only a little bit of liquid with meals** as liquid can dilute the stomach acids required for digestion. Drink liquids at room temperature, if possible. Cold drinks decrease digestive fire.
- **Following your meal, let your body digest the food for fifteen to twenty minutes** before going on to the next activity. Engage in light conversation, read a book, or go for a slow walk. If you are rushed, at least take three to five slow breaths to close the door on this sacred experience.
- **Allow about three hours between meals** for your body to digest. For most people, this means eating three to five meals per day. Do not eat every two to three hours, as many diet plans recommend; this will slow digestion.
- **Breakfast is important.** Please try not to skip it. If you are not hungry in the morning, drink ginger tea to stimulate your appetite and then try to eat. You will find that your appetite for breakfast increases when you eat a smaller, earlier dinner.
- **If possible, eat your largest meal at lunch and the smallest in the evening.** The body's rhythms mirror the rhythms of the universe, and digestion is strongest around noon when the sun is at its peak. Make sure that three hours pass between your last bite of food and bedtime.

BREAKFAST IDEAS

Try these simple, healthy combinations for a good start to your day.

- Cook 1 cup quinoa with ¼ cup sunflower seeds, 2 cups coconut milk, a pinch of salt, ¼ teaspoon ground cardamom, ½ teaspoon ground cinnamon, and ¼ cup blueberries.
- Make chia pudding: Mix 1 cup chia seeds, 2 cups coconut milk, ¼ cup blueberries, ¼ cup chopped pumpkin seeds, a pinch of salt, and ½ teaspoon ground cinnamon in a glass pint jar. Refrigerate overnight and enjoy the next morning.
- Preheat the oven to 425°F. Chop beets, carrots, celery, and parsnips. Toss with olive oil, ground cinnamon, ground coriander, and salt and spread on a baking sheet. Roast for 25 minutes. (You can roast the vegetables ahead of time, if you prefer.) Combine the roasted vegetables with a protein (lentils, a scrambled egg, or cooked chicken).
- Mix 1 cup cooked grain with 1 tablespoon sunflower seed butter or tahini. Add half an avocado and a handful of fresh spinach. Drizzle with lime juice and enjoy.
- Halve an acorn squash and bake it. Scoop out seeds. (You can bake the squash ahead of time, if you prefer.) Smash 2 tablespoons ground hemp seeds into one half of the squash. Sprinkle with ground cinnamon and ground coriander. Reheat in the oven or a toaster oven, if needed. Drizzle with flaxseed oil or olive oil.
- Steam sweet potatoes and kale. Garnish with olive oil, lemon, and sea salt. Enjoy them with two hard-boiled eggs.
- Scramble two eggs with spinach. Serve over leftover roasted root vegetables.
- Sauté ground turkey and chopped spinach in coconut oil with ground cumin, ground coriander, and a bit of ground nutmeg. Top with half an avocado and 1 tablespoon flaxseed meal.
- Top 1 cup cooked quinoa or amaranth with three slices of smoked salmon (check the label to make sure there's no sugar added), a

handful of arugula, and a forkful of sauerkraut (if tolerated). Garnish with a drizzle of flaxseed oil or olive oil.

LUNCH AND DINNER: VARIATIONS OF A SIMPLE "RECIPE"

This recipe is really more of an assembly technique, using a variety of foods that are appropriate for a reset. Eat it for lunch and for dinner. Smaller portions make perfect snacks.

To begin, choose your favorite bowl. It should hold between two and three cups of food. Let this be your eating bowl for the duration of your simplification. Take it with you to work, if necessary.

Prepare the following:

- **Cooked grains.** Choose from the list of appropriate grains above. You might, for example, use buckwheat alone or quinoa mixed with amaranth. Cook them in chicken or beef broth, if you can.
- **Steamed root vegetables.** Chop and steam sweet potatoes, beets, rutabagas or turnips, and carrots.
- **Sautéed greens and/or brassicas.** Chop purple cabbage, chard, and kale. Sauté for ten minutes with olive oil, garlic, a bit of kelp, and salt. Alternatively, you can chop and sauté broccoli, cauliflower, and collard greens.

Now you're ready to eat. Place ⅓ cup of each (grains, roots, greens) in your bowl. Add more grains if you are feeling especially hungry.

Add ⅓ cup of protein (meat, fish, eggs) or 3 tablespoons seeds of your choice. Add more if you are especially active or hungry.

Drizzle with flaxseed or olive oil and lemon juice, and season with salt and pepper.

Garnish your bowl with lacto-fermented vegetables and/or one of these following sauces. You can also use sauce or chutney recipes from other parts of this book.

❧ Carrot Spread

>   5 carrots, diced
>   ¼ cup olive oil
>   1 shallot, minced
>   ¼ teaspoon ground cinnamon
>   ¼ teaspoon ground coriander
>   ¼ teaspoon ground turmeric
>   ¼ teaspoon salt
>   ½ cup chicken or vegetable broth

In a small pot, boil the carrots in water until tender, 12 to 15 minutes. Drain the carrots and set aside to cool.

Combine the oil and minced shallot in a small sauté pan over medium-low heat; sauté for 1 minute, then add the spices and salt. Continue to sauté until the shallots look golden and caramelized, about 5 minutes. Then set aside to cool.

Combine the carrots, shallots, and broth in a blender. Blend until smooth.

❧ Beet Sauce

>   2 medium red beets, sliced in half
>   ¼ cup olive oil
>   1 shallot, minced
>   1 tablespoon apple cider vinegar
>   ½ cup chicken or vegetable broth
>   ¼ teaspoon ground cinnamon
>   ¼ teaspoon ground coriander
>   ¼ teaspoon ground ginger
>   ⅛ teaspoon ground allspice
>   ¼ teaspoon salt

In a small pot, boil the beets in water until tender, about 20 minutes. Once done, drain the beets and set aside to cool.

Combine the oil and minced shallot in a small sauté pan over medium-low heat; sauté for 1 minute, then add the spices and salt. Continue to sauté until the shallots look golden and caramelized, about 5 minutes. Then set aside to cool.

Combine the beets, shallots, vinegar, and broth in a blender. Blend until smooth.

❖ Spinach-Artichoke Sauce

¼ pound spinach
¼ cup olive oil
2 tablespoons tahini (roasted sesame seed butter)
¼ teaspoon salt
1 teaspoon dried thyme
Water as needed to thin the sauce

Place ¼ cup water in a small pot. Add the spinach. Bring to a boil, then reduce the heat to low, cover, and simmer for 2 to 3 minutes. Drain any remaining water.

Drain the artichoke hearts, then put them in a blender with the braised spinach and other ingredients. Blend at the highest speed for 2 minutes. Add water and blend again if you would like the sauce to be thinner.

SNACKS

Here are some of my favorite snacks for you to sample during your reset.

- A hard-boiled egg with olive oil and salt
- 1 tablespoon pumpkin seeds and ¼ cup blueberries
- 1 cup baked sweet potato with 2 tablespoons hemp seeds
- ¼ cup unsweetened coconut yogurt sprinkled with cinnamon
- 1 cup quinoa with ½ avocado and a drizzle of flax oil

The following recipes also make good snack foods.

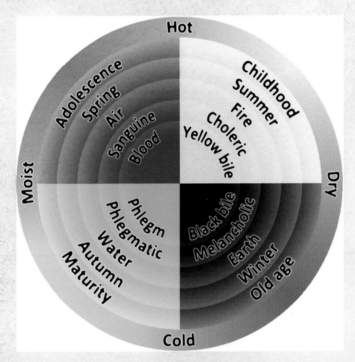

Plate 1. This modern depiction of the humors diagram is based on
models dating back to ancient Greece.
(Courtesy of Royal College of Physicians of Edinburgh.)

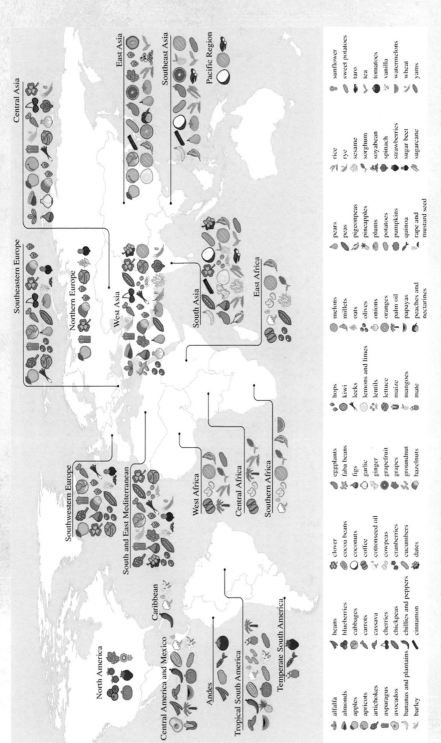

Plate 2. This map from the Royal Society depicts how the origins of food crops connect places around the globe. *(Published by the Royal Society under CC BY 4.0.)*

❧ Quinoa Coconut Pancakes

    1 cup cooked quinoa

    ¼ cup unsweetened shredded coconut

    ¼ cup flaxseed meal

    ½ teaspoon ground cinnamon

    ¼ teaspoon salt

    1½ cups plant milk, plus more as needed

Combine all the ingredients in a large bowl. Mix well. Add a bit more milk if the batter seems too thick. Some milks, like oat milk, are thicker than others. Cook in an oiled skillet as you would cook pancakes.

❧ Whole-Grain Seed Crackers

    ½ cup quinoa, amaranth, or buckwheat

    1½ cups water

    1 cup pumpkin seeds

    1 cup sunflower seeds

    ½ teaspoon salt

    ½ teaspoon dried thyme

    Olive oil

Combine the quinoa, amaranth, or buckwheat with the water in a medium pot. Bring to a boil, then reduce the heat and simmer for about 15 minutes, until the grains have absorbed the water. Transfer the cooked grains to a medium bowl.

    Preheat the oven to 250°F. Grease a baking sheet with olive oil.

    Use a spice/coffee bean grinder to grind the pumpkin and sunflower seeds. Add them to the bowl with the cooked grain and mix well.

    Add the salt and thyme to the bowl and mix well. If mixture seems a bit dry, add a few splashes of olive oil. Be sure that you've mixed well before adding any oil—seeds already contain oil.

    Spread the mixture in a thin layer on the baking sheet.

Bake for I hour. Then turn off the oven and let the cracker tray sit in the oven to cool and crisp up for 5 hours or so.

Let cool completely before breaking into cracker pieces. Store at room temperature in plastic or paper bags.

❧ Coconut Smoothie

I cup fresh or frozen blueberries

I cup full-fat organic coconut milk

I cup water

Juice of ½ lime

¼ cup hemp seeds

2 tablespoons flaxseed meal

¼ teaspoon ground cinnamon

A pinch of salt

Combine all the ingredients in a blender. Blend well and enjoy.

❧ Sushi

I cup quinoa

2 cups water

I tablespoon apple cider vinegar

I teaspoon salt

Vegetables cut into long strips: asparagus, beets, bok
    choy, carrots, daikon radish, scallions, turnips

Nori wrappers

Sesame seeds (optional)

Avocado slices (optional)

Tamari mixed with tahini, for dipping

Combine the quinoa with the water in a small pot. Bring to a boil, then reduce the heat and simmer for about 15 minutes, until the grains have absorbed the water. Stir in the vinegar and salt. Remove from the heat and let cool for 15 minutes.

Meanwhile, steam the vegetables in a simple steamer until just tender (5 minutes or less). Layer the green vegetables on top of the denser root vegetables. Let the vegetables cool for 5 minutes, then start to wrap.

Spread a scoop of cooled quinoa over about one-third of a nori wrapper, along one edge. Make sure that the wrapper's ridges run perpendicular to the quinoa. You will use these ridges as a guide for slicing sections of sushi.

Add a layer of vegetables, followed by sesame seeds and avocado, if desired.

Roll tightly. Moisten the edge of the wrapper with water to press closed.

Slice the roll with a wet knife into six or so sections. Display the sections on a plate.

Repeat the process until you have used all the filling.

Enjoy, dipping the slices into the tamari mixed with tahini.

SUPPORTING THE LIVER

The liver is the source of bile, which is crucial to breaking down food in the stomach. Without the appropriate amount of bile, our metabolic process is greatly affected. Try this simple liver and gallbladder flush for three days to promote liver health and support healthy metabolism.

Upon waking, drink 1 glass warm water with 1 teaspoon lemon juice and 1 teaspoon aloe vera gel.

One hour after lunch, drink a cup of dandelion root tea. Try to drink another one after dinner as well.

Your liver will thank you and your digestion will improve.

BITTERS FOR DIGESTIVE SUPPORT

Another tool for restoring gut health and eliminating cravings is the bitter flavor, which stimulates the natural secretion of digestive enzymes in the upper abdomen. Bitter tastes and flavors also contribute to natural weight loss. Regular exposure to bitter foods in our meals helps promote healthy regeneration of intestinal flora by improving the intestinal environment and disrupting pathogenic germs. These intestinal changes improve the efficiency of our liver, pancreas, and small intestine. Bitters can also help bring our digestion back to normal, improving the elimination of metabolic residues and relieving sensitive digestive tract tissues that can become inflamed by the typical modern Western way of eating.

Bitter foods stimulate the production of digestive fluids and promote complete digestion. They also promote liver detoxification; those with liver and gallbladder issues can benefit from including bitter flavors in meals.

Some examples of bitter foods are amaranth, artichokes, arugula, broccoli, cauliflower, endive, lemons, limes, quinoa, and spices like bay leaf, cardamom, ginger, marjoram, rosemary, sage, and thyme. Many folks enjoy the bitterness of coffee, chocolate, and beer. A bit of these foods can be supportive, but it is easy to overconsume them when we are not including other bitter foods and herbs in our daily eating.

If you do not enjoy bitter foods or wish for extra support from the bitter flavor, try digestive bitters. They keep the enteric brain (the gut brain) from craving sweets and promote bile production for strong digestion. They also can help the pancreas release more digestive enzymes, therefore supporting the absorption of nutrients.

Digestive bitter formulas are an important part of many traditional foodways. In Italy, bitters formulas, or *amari,* are a traditional part of both food culture and cocktail culture. Where my family lives, the two predominant bitters are Alpestre (whose name means Alpine) and Klosterfrau (Cloister Woman). Their recipes have been handed down through regional spiritual practitioners, primarily monks and nuns, for centuries.

TEA BLENDS FOR GUT SUPPORT

A cup of tea offers a wonderful opportunity for a moment of mindfulness. These tea blends are supportive to intestinal motility and gut microbiome balance. As the water comes to a boil, stretch your arms skyward and then reach for your toes. Pour the water over your herbs and sit, watching the steam as the tea steeps.

Store any leftover tea in the fridge to reheat later.

☕ Cumin, Coriander, and Fennel Tea

This traditional Ayurvedic blend of three seeds is digestive, slightly bitter, warming, and balancing. Measure out equal parts of cumin seed, coriander seed, and fennel seed. Bring water to a boil, add the seeds, and simmer, covered, for 15 minutes. (I use 2 tablespoons of each seed and simmer them in 6 cups of water.) Strain and enjoy.

☕ Cinnamon and Licorice Tea

This warming and digestive tea balances blood sugar and has antiviral and immune-boosting properties. Bring 6 cups water to a boil. Add 2 tablespoons chopped licorice root and 1 small cinnamon stick and simmer, covered, for 20 minutes. Strain and enjoy.

☕ Chai

Chai is a Hindi word meaning "tea," and traditionally it is a blend of black tea, cardamom, sugar, and milk. You can make it with any warming spices, like cardamom, cinnamon, cloves, ginger, licorice, and white pepper. Prepare as you would the cinnamon and licorice tea. Strain, add a few tablespoons almond or rice milk, and enjoy!

☕ Lemon Balm Tea

This aromatic herb, whose Latin name is *Melissa officinalis,* is a wonderful antibacterial, digestive, and soothing tea. It calms the nervous system as it stimulates immunity. You can put 2 teaspoons of loose leaf tea in 8 ounces of water and steep for 5 minutes before straining and enjoying.

☕ Tulsi Tea

This herb, also known as sacred basil, is slightly sweet. Tulsi is an adaptogen—an herb that helps us adapt to stress. You can put 2 teaspoons of loose leaf tea in 8 ounces of water and steep for 5 minutes before straining and enjoying.

☕ Marshmallow, Fennel, and Licorice Tea

For those healing from colitis, Crohn's disease, celiac disease, or IBS/IBD, this tea is so healing. Calming and soothing, these herbs help restore the integrity of the intestinal lining and reduce inflammation. I buy them in bulk from the Mountain Rose Herbs online shop. Steep the marshmallow overnight in cold water, then strain, saving the infused water. Bring 3 cups water to a boil. Add 2 tablespoons chopped licorice root and 3 tablespoons fennel seeds and simmer, covered, for 10 minutes. Strain, then combine with the marshmallow-infused water. (Those with hypertension and/or elevated blood pressure, please avoid licorice.)

9

Food Sovereignty

Reclaiming Our Right to Food

Food sovereignty is an affirmation of who we are as indigenous peoples and a way, one of the most surefooted ways, to restore our relationship with the world around us.

WINONA LaDUKE

Winona LaDuke is an Anishinaabe writer and economist from the White Earth lands (colonized name: Minnesota). For her, food sovereignty is about the freedom to choose both what foods to eat and how they were grown. The U.S. Food Sovereignty Alliance, quoting from the Declaration of Nyéléni, the first global forum on food sovereignty, which took place in Mali in 2007, offers the following definition:

Food sovereignty is the right of peoples to healthy and culturally appropriate food produced through ecologically sound and sustainable methods, and their right to define their own food and agriculture systems. It puts the aspirations and needs of those who produce, distribute, and consume food at the heart of food systems and policies rather than the demands of markets and corporations.

Control over land and seeds is an essential part of food sovereignty.

The transnational agrarian movement of small-scale, indigenous farmers known as La Vìa Campesina first spoke of food sovereignty at their second international conference in 1996 in Tlaxcala, Mexico. Peasant farmers gathered there proposed food sovereignty—returning control of land, seeds, water, and natural resources to the indigenous people who grow food—as an alternative to national programs for "food security."

Food sovereignty has been an implicit understanding for people across the globe who live in indigenous foodsheds that have survived for centuries. In the northern Italian region where my family lives, for example, both Austrian and Italian traditions exist, coming together to form a uniquely regional foodshed.

Before World War I, this area was part of the Hapsburg Empire, and though it became part of Italy more than a hundred years ago, it remains ethnically majority Austrian even today. Here, the alpine geography offers only small valleys for habitation, so towns are small and center around churches and farms. Farms feature expansive hay barns with attached stone houses, which hold massive masonry stoves.

Most local people have a working relationship with a few of the farmers in their area. A favorite autumnal pilgrimage involves visiting these farmers for a community meal, with everyone seated at long wooden tables adorned with red-and-white checkered tablecloths. This is such a popular tradition that the name for it, *torgelen,* has become a verb, meaning "to cook and eat together with neighboring farmers." All the shared food is as local as possible. The farmers provide most of it, but the guests bring some too. For a recent farm visit, since the farmer had not collected any berries that season, my aunt Rita made a buttermilk blueberry cake for all to share. Others brought wine from another farmer or a new sausage they had tried while visiting relatives in the Apennine Mountains.

But this is not the end of the community's contribution. When neighbors arrive at the farm in the afternoon, it is time to start cooking. They may be set to work over an open fire, stirring cornmeal, salt, and water in a copper pot with a wooden stick until it thickens into polenta. A farmer might ask for help with slicing thick blocks of speck, a salted and smoked sausage, and displaying them for all to enjoy as appetizers. Some might like to try their hand at rolling out disks of buckwheat flour dough, filling it with steamed spinach and sauerkraut, and folding it into a half-moon shape to make *tirtlen,* large dumplings that are fried and served with plenty of freshly churned butter and Fontina cheese.

Children will run outside, chasing chickens or collecting fallen walnuts to feed to the pigs. Someone in the household might hand out blue aprons embroidered with edelweiss flowers or checkered aprons embroidered with hearts. Guests and farmers alike may tie one on and get to work, tasting wine, roasted chestnuts, speck, and the trademark *schuettelbrot,* a hard rye bread with fennel, fenugreek, and caraway, as the afternoon moves on.

♨ Schuettelbrot

> 1 teaspoon dry yeast
>
> 2 cups water
>
> 3 cups rye flour
>
> 1 cup whole-wheat bread flour, plus a bit for sprinkling hands and work surfaces
>
> 1 teaspoon salt
>
> ¼ teaspoon caraway seeds
>
> ¼ teaspoon fennel seeds
>
> ¼ teaspoon fenugreek seeds

Mix the yeast into ½ cup of the water, stirring to dissolve it. Add 1 cup of the rye flour. Mix until a thick batter forms. Find out where your rye berries came from and who ground them into the flour that will make your bread.

Cover the batter to keep it from drying out and leave it for 30 minutes at room temperature.

Step outside and breathe today's air. There is a lightness to waiting. Perhaps through the clouds you will glimpse the ancestor whose bread baking lives in your deep memories.

Mix the batter with the remaining 1½ cups of water, the remaining 2 cups rye flour, and the whole-wheat flour, salt, and seeds. Cover the dough and allow it to rise until doubled, at least 2 hours, during which my grandmother would boil the soup beans for dinner, walk through the woods for mushrooms, or close her eyes in the pink velvet chair in a dark corner of the living room.

Preheat the oven to 400°F. If you have a bread stone, use it. You can place it on a baking rack in the oven to preheat. If not, bake on a baking sheet.

Divide the dough into two portions. Place them on a well-floured work bench. Flour your hands before handling the dough so that it doesn't stick to you. Coat the dough pieces with flour and let them rest while the oven is heating.

Sprinkle a wooden cutting board (or a baking sheet, if you don't have a board) with flour. Transfer the dough pieces to the board. Shake the board in a circular fashion to make the dough relax and go flat. Imagine a Roma woman, bells jangling from her belt as she dances with the runny dough.

Let the dough pieces rest for 10 minutes.

The loaves will look like circles of dough dotted with healing seeds. Bake them for 15 to 20 minutes, depending on their size.

Once they're done baking, let the loaves cool. Store in a dry place. We wrap ours in brown paper and keep them in the pantry for up to 2 weeks.

By the time the feast is ready, the farmhouse is warm with conversation and the smells of delicious food. From goulash souppe to a winter salad of pickled beets and braised green cabbage to pears poached in red wine, the colors on the table are phenomenal. There is always plenty of bread and wine to go around: baskets and carafes find their way to the table at frequent intervals, heartily refilled by anyone who notices a shortage. By the end of the meal, it is dark. Children are asked to wash a dish or two before all depart, full and satisfied.

⚖ Goulash Souppe

¼ cup olive oil

1 pound grass-fed beef, stew meat, or kebab meat

2 yellow onions, diced

½ cup red wine

1 head garlic, cloves separated, peeled, and chopped

4 stalks celery, chopped

4 carrots, diced

½ teaspoon salt

½ teaspoon freshly ground black pepper

1 tablespoon Hungarian paprika

1 teaspoon dried thyme

½ teaspoon caraway seeds

½ teaspoon cumin seeds

½ teaspoon fenugreek seeds

1 bay leaf

¼ cup tomato paste

4 cups beef broth

Minced fresh parsley, for garnish

Heat the oil in a stock pot over medium heat. Add the beef and onions and sauté until the beef is cooked through, about 5 minutes.

Add the red wine and reduce the heat to low. Add the garlic, celery, and carrots. Add the salt and pepper and stir well. Cook for 15 minutes more. Stretch, read, talk with a loved one, or feed the chickens while you wait. Add a bit of broth if vegetables are sticking to the bottom of the pot.

Add the paprika, thyme, seeds, bay leaf, and tomato paste and stir to incorporate.

Add the broth. Bring to a boil, then reduce the heat and simmer for at least 1 hour and up to 3 hours, depending on the thickness you desire and the chores that might need your attention.

Serve the goulash in bowls while it's still steaming. Sprinkle each bowl with minced parsley. Enjoy with schuettelbrot and good company.

The spirit of collaboration unites people here beyond class and ethnicity. Even though those of Austrian descent are sometimes too proud to send their children to a bilingual school and Italians sometimes resist attending the Austrian folkloric dances that often take place in central squares, everyone can agree about their passion for local food and the picturesque land that makes its growth possible. The tension between two distinct ethnic groups keeps this region vibrant in its struggle, reminding all who live here about the paramount importance of caring for the Earth and appreciating its gifts. Reclaiming control of our food also means reconnecting with the landscape and the people around us as we honor differences and celebrate connection.

In another tradition honored by the local people of the Dolomites, Catholic beliefs twine with the agrarian tradition that came before them. On November 1st, public life stops in Italy. This is All Saints' Day, a celebration of the harvest, an honoring those who have passed, and a connection to the spirit that weaves the seen and unseen worlds together. Gravestones are adorned with purple, red, and yellow chrysanthemums or dried flower arrangements, tall red luminaries, and the love of family members who visit them as they would a living relative. In this tradition the gastronomic and spiritual values of this community unite. Here is my recollection of this special time and one of my first recognitions of the effects of time and modern culture.

When I visit our local church to honor the ancestors, I see the altar adorned in purple satin and covered with baskets of apples, grapes, nuts, cabbages, corn, rye, and buckwheat in thanksgiving for this time of year. A hand-cranked wooden grain thresher, a desk and writing implements, a scythe and felted hat, a pair of dancing shoes, and rows of large pillar candles also decorate the space.

I recognize families who have baked bread, made sausages and wine, and raised goats and chickens in this area for generations. Moving out of the church, the choir intones Gregorian chants as they guide all who are present toward the cemetery atop one of the town's sloping hillsides. Sacred space for the living thrives in the village heart but for those who have passed, the mountain view is more important: it opens a doorway into the next world. On this craggy peak covered mostly in conifers and occasional post-glacial fields people centuries ago managed to erect a chapel with a pointed red steeple, some hay barns and houses, and terraced cultivations. Its ridge is snow-covered already and the rocky Dolomites stand behind it. Tears always spring to my eyes when I see this majestic view and feel the mountain's protection. This is quite a spectacular place to be buried.

As the procession from the church arrives at the cemetery, everyone turns to face their families' graves in prayer. We walk around and around the chapel, honor the Mary and Child inside who are adorned with offerings of food and flowers brought by those who have felt her protection. Walking home, we pass the local monastery and notice that the ancient, twining apple trees in the expansive orchard are laden with fruit. "Why aren't they picking it?" I ask my dad. "There are not many monks left anymore," he replies.

I feel a sadness welling inside me as I realize that this integral human relationship between land, seasons, and prayer belongs to an austere religious tradition that does not appeal to most modern people. However, my young spirit also knows that we do not need to be monks and nuns to grow the food that nourishes us, honor the spirit that binds us, and therefore feed something greater than ourselves. "Let's come back and pick those apples after dark," I suggest. He laughs, nods, and we walk on.

Our family tradition to honor the ancestors then and now involves this simple, rich cake.

✒ Hazelnut Cake

12 ounces hazelnuts

1 teaspoon baking powder

1 teaspoon baking soda

¼ teaspoon salt

6 eggs, separated

½ cup raw honey

½ cup chunky applesauce, unsweetened

Preheat the oven to 325°F.

Grease and flour a 9-inch springform pan. I grew up using olive oil and corn flour to grease and flour pans.

Pour 12 ounces or 12 heaping handfuls of shelled hazelnuts into a food processor or spice grinder.

Grind the hazelnuts until very fine. Add the baking powder, baking soda, and salt. Set aside.

In a large bowl, whip the egg yolks, honey, and applesauce together until smooth. Beat in the ground hazelnut mixture.

In a separate bowl, whisk the egg whites until stiff. Quickly fold 1/3 of the egg whites into the yolk mixture, then add the remaining whites and fold in until no streaks remain.

Pour the batter into the springform pan. Bake in the preheated oven for 60 to 75 minutes, or until the cake springs back when you tap it. Cool it on wire rack.

When the cake is cool, slice it horizontally into 2 layers. Spread the applesauce in between the layers and reassemble the cake. If you would like, you can decorate the top with a thin layer of jam and sprinkle chopped hazelnuts on top.

Serve with espresso after a November Sunday meal.

This weaving of spiritual and physical nourishment of the land and cultures we inhabit is food sovereignty. This link may be what draws people to Italy. It is what keeps the fabric of my homeland's gastronomic traditions alive.

HERITAGE AND FOOD ORIGINS

Today, so much of the world's food has lost its sacred, place-based nature and become a commodity. Many kinds of foods are readily available year-round for those who have the access and privilege to purchase them. However, as plate 2 reveals, the majority of foods that many people consider local staples actually originated in a different place. Apples and garlic originated in Central Asia, while beans and melons come from Africa. Potatoes and tomatoes come from the Andes of South America, while citrus and rice come from Southeast Asia. Oats and cabbage were first found in northern Europe, while carrots and grapes come from the southern Mediterranean.

The more we eat in accordance with our heritage, the more we feel balanced. This process may involve looking at aspects of our inheritance that are hard to see and offering them forgiveness so that we can continue the work of promoting equity. The more we eat in accordance with the foods native to the regions in which we live, the better we align ourselves with our environment and, again, the more we lean into feeling balanced. At the same time, the more we learn about the foodways of local indigenous peoples, the more we learn to appreciate and respect the wisdom of traditional cultures. In this way, eating becomes an opportunity to re-localize: to honor our ancestors, our environment, our communities, everything that has brought us to this moment, and to achieve well-being while doing so.

Reverence for local foods can be found in many places worldwide. My experience of being raised in the Mediterranean climate is that it allows food traditions to shine through the variety of ingredients available year-round. Where I live now on unceded Abenaki land in Vermont, farmers cultivate beautiful vegetables, tend to winter-hardy fruit trees, pasture healthy animals, and grow an impressive variety of grains. But our growing season lasts five months at best, and as our supplies of local foods dwindle during the cold months, so does my desire grow to visit the warmer places where these foods grow year-round.

Certain parts of California may reflect the Italian peninsula's growing season, but food grown at that scale does not compare to the small production to which Italy must adhere due to its mountainous geography. With the Apennines running a spine north–south and the Alps holding the northern part of the country, there are few places to cultivate anything on more than a handful of acres. Hence, even though the growing season here is luxurious, Italian food acquires a precious quality due to its small-scale production. Regional recipes are integral to the cultural paradigm. Each region of Italy is distinct and specific in its culinary traditions. Our family enjoys our own and cooks from others as well. This way, we learn and honor our neighbors.

When I was growing up, my family loved a meal of pomegranate risotto and roast rabbit with white wine and chestnuts. To make the beloved *primo piatto,* or first course, with the tangy, crimson-seeded fruit that informs the length of Persephone's stay in the underworld, it is essential to remove the seeds from the fruit body, boil them briefly, and spin them through a sieve to catch the brilliant juice. This succus becomes part of the broth in which we cook the rice.

We also enjoyed roasted rabbit with white wine and chestnuts. Rabbit meat is rich and lean but often has a gamey flavor unless retained water is first removed by searing and then rinsing the rabbit. So first, we seared and rinsed the rabbit to remove the gamey flavor before placing it in a roasting pan. We'd make a paste of garlic and dried rosemary and sage we'd collected when we visited the hill village Arquà Petrarca and use it to coat the rabbit and help it to retain its juices while roasting. We'd pour a quarter bottle of the white wine made by one of my father's university colleagues into the roasting pan and send it on its way into the hot oven.

Meanwhile, we sliced crescents along the rinds of chestnuts gleaned from Imperia, a nearby town on the ocean. We placed them on a baking sheet and roasted them until the nut meat began to escape from each sliced section. We would want to peel them immediately and savor their sweetness as a prelude to our meal, but we had to allow them to cool. Instead, we sampled some of the rye bread we had baked with flour from my family's hometown in the Dolomite mountains, alongside a few of the tangy, tiny black olives that my father picked and pickled in Pienza, Tuscany, the previous autumn. Bread and olives can provide enough temporary respite to any hungry Italian. Later, when we added the chestnuts to the rabbit and gave the risotto its final stir and last drizzle of olive oil, we could sit down to dinner satisfied by the process before even taking our first bite.

Every spring, we made egg-basted asparagus in the traditional way that my father learned from his grandmother while living with her during World War II. As the trees put on leaves and dandelion decorated the forest edges, chickens would start laying eggs just as asparagus pushed its way through the earth, making itself available to provide nourishment and prebiotic benefit after a long winter without green vegetables.

Papi Mi Ha Insegnato

"Luzellette mi ha insegnato." Papi would explain
how she had taught him to dig under fallen oak leaves
for morels after spring rain, to scour southern slopes
for boletes and chantrelles once summer solstice waned,
to respect the fierce red amanitas and let them go by.
Papi and I decide to make egg-basted asparagus,
a recipe from great-grandmother Luzellette,
Little Bird, who lived and died in Gaby,
near an alpine stream that bouldered down
the steep slopes she walked with pack basket
and sickle to harvest fresh grass for her goats.
Nothing but goat milk, potatoes, and polenta
in those war years. He learned not to get kicked
while milking, to leave milk in the stone house,
where it waited for hungry neighbors
who had sold their animals for flour.
We cook the asparagus recipe so it will not
be forgotten, told every time it is prepared

to honor the first truth of green spears
finding their way through black dirt, earth arrows
that we gather and steam before they grow
delicate fronds that make seeds like tiny globes.

✒ Egg-Basted Asparagus

Olive oil

About 15 spears asparagus

Salt and freshly ground black pepper

4 eggs

1 tablespoon stone-ground mustard

Preheat the oven 400°F. Oil a square baking dish with olive oil.

Snap the ends off the asparagus and lay the tender spears in the baking dish in a criss-cross pattern. Sprinkle with salt and pepper. Bake for 10 minutes.

Whisk the eggs and mustard together. Stir in a pinch of salt.

Remove the asparagus from the oven and drizzle it with the whisked egg mixture.

Bake for 10 minutes more, until the eggs are just set.

Garnish with olive oil and enjoy.

RELOCALIZING FOOD

[Food sovereignty] is a call for the right of everyone to be able actively to shape the food system, rather than being shaped by it. It's a call for a democratic debate and action around food, and about redistributing power more equitably in the food system.

RAJ PATEL

When I lived on the island of Bali in 2000, I found myself sharing space with a group of people whose food sovereignty had been taken from them during the Green Revolution of the 1960s and '70s. Most Balinese rice was exported, while the Balinese people ate high-yield, genetically modified rice imported from other parts of Asia. The Indonesian government also forced them to grow this new rice and to flood their traditional *subaks,* sacred irrigation systems directed by priests, with pesticides. (Even today, many Balinese people are still fighting the impacts of these impositions, and they are slowly gaining ground. There are now multiple World Heritage sites on Bali where locals are growing rice in the traditional way and saving the seeds to assert sovereignty.)

The Balinese with whom I lived focused on what they could control: the wildcrafting of fruits such as coconut and spices such as galangal. I learned to cook with coconut oil, a plant-based saturated fat and the only food other than breast milk that is high in lauric acid. This high-quality fatty acid is indigenous to the Indonesian archipelago and exhibits anti-inflammatory and antimicrobial properties.[1] Its use in local cuisine protects the digestive tract from the bacteria and fungi that are common in this tropical environment.

When people consider a food sacred, they use all parts of it. In Bali, after the coconut flesh is pressed for oil, it is blended with the liquid inside to create coconut milk, a creamy substance rich in potassium, magnesium, and amino acids. The coconut milk is eaten with green vegetables and low-fat protein, such as tempeh, which allows the body to process the coconut's medium-chain fatty acids and effectively use them for energy instead of storing them as fat.

Although those who, like families I lived with on Bali, still center their eating around indigenous foods and cultural foodways comprise the global majority, they do not have access to the same privileges as colonists in Europe, the United States, and Canada. The imbalance created by white supremacy culture and colonial capitalism has led to the need for a new approach to food systems, one founded in equity, climate resiliency, and equal access to land and culturally appropriate, whole foods for all. According to the United Nations, "When transformed with greater resilience to major drivers, including conflict, climate variability and extremes, and economic slowdowns and downturns, food systems can provide affordable healthy diets that are sustainable and inclusive, and become a powerful driving force towards ending hunger, food insecurity and malnutrition in all its forms, for all."[2]

Supporting food sovereignty can play an important role in building resilience into food systems. And there's a huge need for it. Hunger and lack of access to land and food remain tremendous issues across the globe. In a 2021 report, the Food and Agriculture Organization of the United Nations noted that "between 720 and 811 million people in the world faced hunger in 2020" and predicted that "around 660 million people may still face hunger in 2030."[3]

As Ana Moragues Faus, a professor of agricultural economics at the University of Barcelona, says:

> Resilience and regeneration are not a given, they need to be purposefully nurtured. We therefore need to facilitate the creation of food systems based on local needs and capacities that assure a fair redistribution of value, knowledge, and power across actors and territories to deliver sustainable food for all.[4]

Food sovereignty, Moragues Faus explains, is a tool to relocalize the food system, make democracy accessible to all, care for community, and respect the intersectionality of all ancestral foodways. In our modern world, we must work to harmonize the ancestral foods that live inside of us with the local foods of the communities in which we now live. Most of my cousins still live in my hometown in the Dolomites. I have traveled to live in a similar climate but on a different continent. This shift requires attention, both to my changing needs and to the indigenous foods of my current landscape.

Because I grew up in a place where food acts as a unifier and equalizer, I have always valued stepping away from corporate, processed food and putting resources toward local, culturally appropriate food. I see this practice as a crucial step in ensuring food sovereignty for all people. What does it look like for you to understand the indigenous food traditions of your ancestors and your community as a way to regain control over your food? Can you connect with local farmers and other producers and get your food from them? Do you want to join a community garden or expand your own garden? Can you set up a seasonal food swap with friends and neighbors? Can you support indigenous peoples' struggles to regain and maintain control of their ancestral lands and seeds?

One of the ways I practice food sovereignty in my daily life is to take a more intuitive approach to cooking. I substitute ingredients because I am learning about their origins and their nutrient content. I strive to honor the sacredness of all food as I weave different ingredients into meals. Cooking is a creative process. The more we understand how ingredients relate to each other, the more aligned our dishes will become, both with our needs and with the planet's need to relocalize the food system for the sake of survival.

Cooking creatively, using what's available locally, can support an intuitive eating practice and the desire to understand and respect the roots of the dishes you prepare. The more we listen to the body's requests for specific foods, the more we learn how to prepare meals that can be more enjoyable for us in a particular moment in time. For me, recipes are suggestions, not strict rules. Traditional people, including my Italian grandmother, would only ever pass down a recipe orally. The first time I cooked millet with twice as much liquid as the recipe suggested, I created a creamy, polenta-like porridge. I found that I enjoyed millet more in this form. As we start to develop comfort with doing so, cooking from a place of creativity and intuition allows us to incorporate different seasonal ingredients and substitute based on budget as well, thus taking control of our nourishment from the inside out.

LEARNING FROM THE DINÉ

As a college student, I had the privilege of spending a semester studying abroad on Diné tribal land at Diné College. During our studies of traditional Diné culture, language, pottery, and creation story, a fellow student and I lived through profound experiences. We learned that Diné culture is animist and committed to dual inequality, meaning that everything is alive and that life is a constant practice of creating imbalance and restoring balance. This principle is elucidated through the words *Są́'a Naghái Bik'eh Hózhó*. Because the Diné language is vibrational, it echoes the sounds of nature. I am not a Diné person, so I cannot accurately translate these words, but they can be understood as the vibrations that restore balance, also known as the Beauty Way, which creates reality through the spiritual intention placed in the spoken word.

Without imbalance, there is no opportunity to create balance. Without challenges from other groups of people, such as the Ancestral Pueblo or Spanish and English colonists, Diné culture lacks the opportunity to restore the Beauty Way. Through these teachings, I learned to embrace conflict to gain resolution. Chinese medicine would refer to this concept as "going with the flow." When we resist conflict, it grows in opposition to the resistance. Instead, embracing it dissolves it. This is the foundational healing concept of the Diné Blessingway Ceremony. If illness is imbalance, or conflict, a patient must commune with the conflict to heal. When we try to medicate illness, we infuse the body with more conflict, which ultimately leads to side effects and additional illnesses.

Without embracing the difficulty of being a white colonist on native land, I would not have had the opportunity to learn what it means to listen to and respect the needs of others. I would not have had the opportunity to embrace that conflict, not take it personally, and gain resolution through the power of sacred language and ceremony.

Understandably, it took some time for us to be accepted into the community. We clearly were not Diné, yet we had been allowed to study there thanks to friendships between professors. The other students called us the vanilla ice cream girls, and rightfully so. We understood when the students who were meant to share a bathroom with us asked to be moved to another dormitory. White-skinned colonists need to learn how to listen to the global majority. We received this message loud and clear during our time on Diné land.

Over the course of months, we learned how to keep the pack of local dogs from following us around campus and snarling at us. We even befriended one who slept outside our window every night and ate the containers of taco meat that we brought her from the cafeteria. Eventually, students stopped hissing at us when we walked past, and some even began to talk with us. With patience, we finally forged connections with some Diné students, particularly those who had previously spent time off the reservation, primarily in the military, and had befriended other white folks during their time away. Thanks to their kindness, we were invited to attend a Native American Church ceremony.

Today, it might not be possible to have the honor of experiencing what we did then, in the fall of 1999. Part of honoring traditional cultures that have been oppressed and even erased is the solemn agreement not to share their traditions—that is their privilege alone. I will simply offer that the experience of sitting overnight in a tipi with drum, song, fire, and the sacred medicine of the peyote cactus was life changing. It connected me to the Earth and taught me that I am a part of nature in a way that no other plant medicine experience ever had.

When we stepped outside the tipi to greet the dawn, there was mutton stew and bread ready for everyone. We grounded back to our bodies thanks to the gift of traditional nourishment. We were held by the tribal community thanks to the connective power of the medicine.

Preparing and eating traditional indigenous foods is an integral part of the sacred rituals and ceremonies that anchor the Diné to their identity and their survival. Despite the invasion of corporate, processed food, the Diné have been able to keep their culinary traditions alive as a tool to restore the Beauty Way, Sa'a Naghái Bik'eh Hózhó, in their lives. Their sense of sovereignty is essential to maintaining and uplifting the cultural traditions that weave together the sacred reality in the indigenous worldview.

SEEDS OF RENEWAL

When Fred Wiseman bit into one of the ground cherries he had just purchased at a farm stand in Hardwick, his taste buds suddenly sparked memories of his grandmother's cooking. "She made ground cherry sauce and served it over fish," he explained to me. "I was a kid and I didn't like it. There were too many seeds." This kind of recollection, along with many others from Abenaki people in this bioregion, has shaped the tribe's struggle for recognition and its subsequent revival of indigenous agricultural, culinary, and ceremonial practices. Professor Wiseman is an ethnobotanist, native rights advocate, and Abenaki tribal member. In 2012, he launched the Seeds of Renewal project to encompass the full spectrum of a sovereign Abenaki food system, from seed-saving and farming to the development of a cookbook and a seed bank by and for tribal members. He has been working tirelessly to track down and reintroduce original crops and cultivation methods to Abenaki gardeners and farmers.

For indigenous people, "identity is a negotiation between who I say I am and who society says I am," Wiseman mused. This project not only returns traditional seeds and foods to native people, but it also helps others see the Abenaki for who they are. This is food sovereignty: the connection between insider and outsider that uplifts the food traditions that are sacred.

The Seeds of Renewal project took root soon after the Abenaki tribe gained Vermont state recognition. After interviewing many Abenakis to support the case for recognition, Professor Wiseman noticed similarities in peoples' stories. He realized that many local indigenous people connect their tribal identity to agriculture.

Through a career of ethnobotanical research with the Hopi people in Arizona and the Mayo and Yaqui peoples in northwestern Mexico, Wiseman had gained a profound appreciation for these groups' self-identification. During our conversations he explained, "Agriculture is the engine of identity for these tribes. They see themselves as the keepers of the land, crops, and spirituality that connects them." When he returned to northern Vermont to care for his mother, he began to question how his own ancestors saw themselves.

Wiseman said he had previously misunderstood traditional Abenaki agriculture as employing a basic "slash and burn" technique. Because records and firsthand accounts were missing, he started talking with indigenous elders. They recounted stories of a different kind of farming, one that was complex, connected to seasonal ritual, and reflective of people who identify agriculturally. He listened and realized that these stories reflected indigenous farming practices recorded by French explorer Samuel de Champlain in the early seventeenth century.

Nancy Doucet, chief of the Koasek band of the Koas Abenaki Nation, told Wiseman that their ancestors had their own variety of corn, and they had given it to white colonists in the 1790s. She told him about a Vermont farming family that had kept the seed pure and recently returned it to the Abenaki. He was astounded. Not only were his people agriculturally sophisticated, but they still had access to their seeds. The seed chase began.

Crops such as the rare and endangered Gaspé and Abenaki Rose corn, skunk beans, and Algonquin squash have a long history of being grown by indigenous people of the region but are becoming rare. Thanks to Professor Wiseman's research and Peggy Fullerton's propagation at the Koasek farm near Newbury, Vermont, these traditional seeds are being grown with the traditional mound system.

As Peggy explained to Wiseman, "The Koasek garden, named Sagakwa, is 40 feet by 200 feet. Down the road, we have a separate plot to grow vegetables that cross pollinate. In case a crop fails in one location, seed is grown in tribe members' personal gardens. Our original Koasek corn has been growing here since 2006. We have plans to expand and produce even more food for members of the tribe, elders in our villages, local senior centers, and any canning and preserving needs."

Food sovereignty respects the right for all people to define their own food systems from the ground up and honors all participants of every food system equally. "It is essential to educate others about the traditional seeds and honor the native people who have grown and saved them," Cheryl O'Neil explained during our conversations. She is a gardener at the Abenaki Heritage Garden at the Intervale Center in Burlington, Vermont, and an Abenaki tribe member. Her background in health care inspires her to educate others about the importance of eating local food that's grown and prepared in a wholesome way. She believes that "we are all the Creator's people. We need to get others on board with eating simple, wholesome food." First, they must grow out the seeds for multiple years to have enough stock. Thanks to the efforts of Seeds of Renewal project, O'Neil's dream to taste her own native corn and share it with others is becoming a reality.

Through the project's continued efforts, Abenakis can maintain their indigenous agricultural, spiritual, and culinary traditions. Funding and additional research are required to confirm the genetics and nutritional value of these indigenous crops. Meanwhile, Professor Wiseman and his cohorts continue their work. The recipes below provide a taste of an extensive compendium that has been revived through the project.

🌶 Cheryl's Summer Succotash

> 1 cup Vermont cranberry beans or Marfax beans
> 4 ears fresh corn
> 4 tablespoons butter
> Salt and freshly ground black pepper
> Chopped fresh parsley, for garnish

Soak the beans in water for 8 hours or overnight. Then drain and rinse.

Combine the beans in a pot with 4 cups water. Bring to a boil, then reduce the heat and simmer for about 40 minutes, or until beans are tender. Drain. One cup of dried beans will yield 2 cups of cooked beans.

Meanwhile, cut the corn kernels off the cobs. Scrape the milk off the cobs into a bowl by using the back of a knife or a spoon.

Melt the butter in a deep skillet over medium heat. Add the corn kernels, corn milk, and salt and pepper to taste. Cook for 5 minutes, stirring often.

Add the beans and cook for 5 more minutes. Taste, and add more salt and pepper if you wish. Serve warm, garnishing each bowl with chopped parsley.

Recipe courtesy of Koasek band member Cheryl O'Neil

✕ Nancy's Summer Soup

2 cups hominy

2 cups green beans

2 cups peeled, cubed summer squash

1½ cups peeled, diced potatoes

5 cups water

2 tablespoons chicken or vegetable bouillon

2 tablespoons flour

2 tablespoons butter, melted

½ teaspoon freshly ground black pepper

Place the hominy, green beans, squash, and potatoes into a pot. Pour in the water and bouillon. Bring to a boil, then reduce the heat to low and simmer until the vegetables are soft, about 10 minutes.

Blend the flour into the melted butter, then stir the mixture into the soup. Increase heat to medium and cook until the soup thickens.

Season with pepper and serve.

A specialty of Nancy Doucet, the late chief of the Koasek of the Koas

10

Starting Your Culinary Pharmacy

Staple Foods and Their Benefits

Thirty years of nutritional advice have left us fatter, sicker, and more poorly nourished. Which is why we find ourselves in the predicament we do: in need of a whole new way to think about eating.

MICHAEL POLLAN

Ancestral foods are our birthright. We each have genetic programming that informs the ideal way of eating for us. Environment and circumstances can alter our food choices as we move through life, but the life-giving nourishment of our ancestors is a touchstone for restoring balance time and time again. I found this to be true when healing myself from chronic infection, childbirth, and autoimmune thyroid disease. May we all find ways to remember ancestral superfoods in our daily eating rhythms.

When we learn about "superfoods" from other parts of the world and start selling them on the American health food market, the effect is often devastating to the people who rely on the foods that are indigenous to them. As examples, the sudden popularity of amaranth led to an amaranth crisis in Oaxaca, Mexico, in the 1970s, while Bolivia is currently recovering from a quinoa crisis.

Amaranth is the primary food for lactating mothers in Oaxaca because it prevents candida yeast overgrowth, supports breast milk production, and is loaded with essential amino acids. Quinoa is essential for Andean villagers who must walk between places that are at high altitudes, providing endurance fuel while also relaxing the muscles with its high magnesium content so that people do not get sore after walking many miles each day.

When you become interested in a food that's not local to you, find out where it comes from. Talk with local farmers to see whether they might be able to grow it. By becoming involved in our local food systems, we can allow other people to maintain control of theirs.

A food's origins speak both to our ancestral connection with it and to the interconnections of groups of people. The iconic schuettelbrot, hard rye bread with fennel, fenugreek, and caraway, that is traditional in the Dolomite mountains of my homeland, contains spices that traveled from India and the Fertile Crescent with merchants and nomads before becoming part of my ancestral traditions. Fenugreek's name comes from the Latin *foenum graecum*, meaning "Greek hay"; Romans used it as cow feed. In the Greco-Roman healing tradition, it is also used to heal the lungs and the large intestine. This little seed, a member of the leguminous pea family, came to Greece via Africa, Iran, and Iraq. It features prominently in dishes and spice blends from Ethiopia and Sudan.

My family eats schuettelbrot doused in olive oil to soften it, enhance its flavor, and add the fat necessary to properly digest the carbohydrates contained in rye flour. Olive oil is a sacred food, a fruit oil, and one that I learned so much about when I helped family friends with their harvest. Their grove of three hundred olive trees lines the slopes of Monticchiello in the Val d'Orcia region of southern Tuscany. Olive trees thrive here in clay soil so thick that it would routinely pull off my muck boots as I walked down the rows, shaking olives from branches into the nets that we had laid out below. I would simply shove a now-muddy sock back into my boot and carry on: we had to gather the olive-filled nets, dump them into crates, and haul the crates to the press inside the walled town of Pienza by nightfall so that they would not go rancid. After visiting the press and returning home with our precious oil, we would feast until midnight on prosciutto, artichokes, and *pici con aglione,* a traditional Tuscan pasta dish. After a heartfelt toast with limoncello, our harvesting team would go to sleep and do it all over again the next day.

Working in partnership with the land to enjoy the sacred foods to which we owe our lives is not easy. When a bottle of olive oil makes its way to your kitchen, think of the long days of patient labor required to gain that green gold. The Benedictine monks coined the phrase *ora et labora,* "pray and work." If work means paying attention to what is sacred in any given moment, then it certainly applies to the process of harvesting olives to make olive oil.

Every food and herb that lives in harmony with humans has a story of how it has traveled and influenced cuisine and health. Fenugreek is just one example of an ancestral food that connects many different traditions and ancestral foodways.

Use this culinary medicine guide as a starting point for determining which ancestral foods resonate in your body, mind, and spirit.

FATS

Note: I have included nuts and seeds in this category because they are an excellent source of healthy fats. They are intersectional foods, though, and also contain protein and fiber.

Any nut is more digestible when it is soaked overnight and then dehydrated in the oven. I usually bake soaked nuts at 300°F for 30 minutes.

Almonds
These tree nuts are high in monounsaturated fat, which promotes heart health, helps reduce LDL cholesterol, and aids in carbohydrate metabolism. Almonds contain flavoproteins to balance blood sugar and

improve energy levels. They are rich in vitamin E to promote cognitive health and protect the brain from oxidative stress. In Ayurveda, almonds are touted as a rejuvenation tonic that builds *ojas,* life force energy, which is known as *jing* in Chinese medicine. They have a bittersweet flavor.

Coconut Oil

A saturated fat, coconut oil is a plant-based alternative to butter. It contains medium-chain fatty acids that help reduce stress and prevent depression. It stimulates brain function and promotes intestinal motility. It is antibacterial, making it an important food to choose during times of illness or infection. It is specifically indicated for combating intestinal parasites and candida yeast overgrowth. Its lauric acid content makes it an excellent skin tonic, and it can be applied topically to sooth dry skin, eczema, or psoriasis. Coconut oil is cooling and sweet.

Ghee

Ghee, or clarified butter, is unsalted butter that has been separated from its water and milk proteins (see recipe, page 33). Ghee is rich in vitamins A, E, and K, which are crucial for overall health. It also contains CLA (conjugated linoleic acid), which assists the body in burning stored fat, and butyric acid, a short-chain fatty acid that supports colon health. It has a high smoke point, which makes it ideal for cooking at high heat. Ghee is warming, sweet, and rich.

Olive Oil

First cold-press olive oil is a monounsaturated fat that is high in anti-inflammatory polyphenols, which support heart health, help maintain balanced cholesterol, and reduce the overgrowth of ulcer-inducing *Helicobacter pylori* bacteria in the small intestine. It helps increase calcium levels in the blood and enhances memory function by oxygenating blood. Olive oil is warming and primarily bitter, though it has some pungent notes as well. (See page 50 for details on olive oil classifications and labeling.)

Peanuts

These legumes are a good source of anti-inflammatory vitamin E, niacin for brain health, folate, protein, manganese, and resveratrol, the phenolic antioxidant that lowers blood pressure and promotes heart health. Make sure to always eat them roasted for maximum digestibility and health benefit. They also contain beta-sitosterols, which help the nervous system shift into parasympathetic rest mode. Peanuts can be difficult to digest because of their high fat content. They are rich, sweet, and salty.

Sesame Seeds

Sesame seeds promote elasticity of bones and joints with their vitamin E content. They are rich in calcium for healthy metabolism and bone density. They also help the colon extract water from food waste before elimination occurs. Cuneiform tablets from the Fertile Crescent contain writing about these tiny seeds dating back to 3500 BCE. They are indigenous to both India and Ethiopia and have traveled with merchants for centuries to reach other parts of the world. A common preparation is tahini, or sesame seed butter. Sesame seeds are bitter and a bit sour.

Sunflower Oil

This polyunsaturated oil is rich in vitamin E, which stimulates liver rejuvenation and aids in nutrient absorption. Its high magnesium content soothes nerves and muscles, acts as a diuretic to counteract water retention, and lubricates the digestive system to aid elimination. Sunflower oil is warming, slightly bitter, unctuous, and sweet.

Sunflower Seeds

These power-packed seeds contain selenium to detoxify the liver and blood, help DNA repair itself, and support thyroid function; magnesium to strengthen bones, calm nerves, and support immunity; vitamin E to protect cells with its anti-inflammatory effects; and phytosterols to reduce overall blood cholesterol. They are a good source of protein and unsaturated fat. Sunflower seeds taste unctuous, pungent, and bitter.

Walnuts

Walnuts are rich in omega-3 essential fatty acids and ellagic acid, which supports the immune system. They contain vitamin E as gamma-tocopherol, which helps maintain heart health, and are slightly laxative. Their high tannin content gives them a characteristic bitter flavor, but they also have a sweet character, especially after being soaked and baked.

FRUITS AND VEGETABLES

Apples

These fall fruits contain polyphenols and fiber to help maintain balanced blood glucose. They also contain prebiotic compounds that feed intestinal flora and ease gas and bloating. Apples contain antioxidants that support the breakdown of dietary fats and reduce the risk of cardiovascular difficulties. The fructo-oligosaccharides in apples can make them challenging to digest when raw. Cooked apples are easier on the digestive system. Apples are cooling, sweet, and a bit sour.

Artichokes

These spring and summer vegetables help with the digestion of fat due to their capacity to support the liver. Artichokes balance an overly acidic stomach. They strengthen vision, bones, and joints due to their magnesium, calcium, and vitamin C content. They also contain cynarin, a phytonutrient that supports healthy bile production in the liver. They are neutral, slightly bitter, and sour.

Asparagus

Rich in prebiotic compounds that nourish beneficial intestinal bacteria, asparagus also has high levels of antioxidants such as vitamin C, vitamin E, and glutathione, which reduce inflammation. It also contains flavonoids such as quercetin that are antiviral and reduce blood pressure. Asparagus has high levels of insoluble fiber, which promotes healthy, regular bowel movements. Asparagus is cooling, bitter, and sour.

Avocado and Avocado Oil

Rich in carotenoids and B vitamins, anti-inflammatory agents that lubricate muscles and joints, avocados also support cardiovascular health and help balance blood glucose. They are also high in oleic acid, a monounsaturated fat that promotes satiety, and beta-sitosterol, a plant sterol that benefits both the nervous system and the cardiovascular system. Avocados contain folate, which helps remove homocysteine buildup in the system that can contribute to mood imbalances. They are rich and slightly sweet.

Beets

Beets are an excellent source of phytonutrients called betalains, which provide antioxidant, anti-inflammatory, and liver detoxification support. They are rich in manganese and vitamin C, which promote nervous system health, and also high betaine, an essential nutrient made from choline. Choline reduces inflammation in the cardiovascular system by preventing unwanted buildup of homocysteine, an inflammatory compound. Beets are in the amaranth family (along with amaranth, chard, quinoa, and spinach), and their high oxalate levels could be harmful to those with kidney challenges. Beets are neutral, earthy, and sweet.

Blueberries

These berries are anti-inflammatory, antioxidant, and rich in anthocyanins, plant compounds that are associated with brain and nervous system function, specifically with improving memory and reducing depression. Blueberries are low on the glycemic index, making them ideal for those with insulin resistance, metabolic syndrome, or diabetes. They are cooling, sweet, and detoxifying.

Burdock Root

This milky root is cooling and tonic. It relieves dry skin, strengthens hair follicles, stimulates appetite, and cleanses the liver. It is supportive to the lungs and large intestine. Peel it, rinse it, chop it, and sauté it as you would a carrot. It is also delicious simmered in soup. Burdock is cooling, bitter, and slightly pungent.

Cabbage, Purple/Red

A cruciferous vegetable in the brassica family, cabbage contains polyphenols, cancer-preventive phytonutrients. High in vitamins A and C to boost immunity, cabbage is also rich in glucosinolates, which reduce inflammation and help heal stomach ulcers. It cools summer heat and reduces fevers and topical infections. Place cabbage leaves on a wound or infection, such as mastitis, to draw heat from the affected area. Cabbage is neutral, sweet, and pungent.

Carrots

These root vegetables are high in nutrients that are essential for eye health: beta-carotene, lutein, and zeaxanthin. Beta-carotene can also help stop damage to DNA and reduce the risk of clogged arteries. Carrots contain many plant nutrients that are both antioxidant and supportive to immune health, including vitamin C and polyphenols, among others. They contain both soluble and insoluble fiber to support intestinal motility and beneficial gut bacteria. Carrots are slightly bitter and mostly sweet.

Cauliflower

A cruciferous vegetable in the brassica family, cauliflower is high in vitamin C and manganese, two antioxidant nutrients. It supports the body's daily detoxification process and contains vitamin K to support blood clotting, bone density, and calcium balance. It strengthens weak or sluggish digestion. Cauliflower is neutral, sweet, and bitter.

Dandelion Root

Dandelion root helps cleanse the digestive system, improves elimination, and relieves gassiness, especially in the spring. It is a gentle liver and gallbladder tonic and is slightly diuretic. Peel and chop two tablespoons of root per pint of soup stock or sauté it with tempeh for an earthy breakfast delight. Dandelion root is cooling, sweet, and bitter.

Dark Leafy Greens

Collards and kale, members of the brassica family, are rich in folic acid and calcium. They contain glucosinolates, which support liver detoxification and nourish intestinal flora with their prebiotic compounds. All brassica family plants (including broccoli and cabbage) provide 85 percent of our recommended daily fiber intake in just 200 calories (about five servings). Collards and kale also help prevent overgrowth of *Helicobacter pylori*, which can lead to digestive disturbances such as IBS and colitis. These greens are warming, sweet, and bitter.

Garlic

High in vitamin C and pungent sulfurous compounds, which reduce inflammation in the body, garlic is nature's most potent antibiotic. It contains polysulfides, which trigger blood vessel dilation to reduce blood pressure. It controls overgrowth of *Helicobacter pylori* in the small intestine, thus helping to reduce heartburn and eventual ulcers. Garlic is very warming as well as slightly sweet and pungent.

Leeks

Like other members of the allium family (onions, garlic, shallots, scallions), leeks are antimicrobial and antibacterial. They are rich in fructo-oligosaccharides, which stimulate the growth of healthy intestinal bacteria and suppress the growth of potentially harmful bacteria in the colon. Leeks are warming, sour, sweet, and pungent.

Mushrooms

These members of the fungal kingdom have a rich, earthy flavor and are relatively high in protein. In addition, they are anti-inflammatory, immune-boosting, and antioxidant. They also contain CLA (conjugated linoleic acid), which may be able to bind onto aromatase enzymes in breast cancer cells and lessen their ability to produce estrogen. Mushrooms are neutral, earthy, and sweet.

Nettles

Warming and drying, this spring plant helps ease water retention, supplies iron and other minerals, and detoxifies the system that's prone to seasonal allergies. Pick the young leaves carefully, as they can sting. Steam them so that they no longer sting and add them to your favorite vegetable dish. Nettles have a sour, bitter flavor.

Onions

Like other members of the allium family (leeks, garlic, shallots, scallions) onions are anti-microbial and anti-bacterial. They are rich in prebiotic fiber that feeds beneficial gut bacteria for stronger digestion and immunity. Onions are sour, sweet, and pungent.

Pears

Pears are loaded with flavanols, plant nutrients that provide anti-inflammatory and antioxidant support, and also rich in pectin, a sugar high in galacturonic acid, which coats and soothes the intestines to reduce symptoms of heartburn, ulcers, GERD, acid reflux, and colitis. Pear fibers bind with bile acid in the intestines, making them easily digestible. They are unctuous and sweet.

Raspberries

These berries have anticancer and anti-inflammatory properties. They provide excellent support for cognitive function, memory, and mood. They contain ellagic acid, which is associated with potentially inhibiting the development of various cancers and with destroying the human papilloma virus (HPV) responsible for cervical cancer. Resveratrol, present in raspberries, red wine, cocoa powder, and peanuts, has been shown to help inhibit Alzheimer's and Parkinson's diseases. Raspberries are sour-sweet in flavor.

Rutabagas and Turnips

These close relatives are members of the cruciferous brassica family. These root vegetables support the production of digestive secretions with their bitter and pungent flavor and cleanse the intestines of mucus buildup. They are mostly pungent, although rutabagas are slightly sweet and turnips are bitter.

Sea Vegetables

Anti-inflammatory, antiviral, and rich in minerals, seaweeds promote healthy brain function and help clear heavy metals from the system. They are high in iodine, which helps regulate thyroid hormone production. Choose nori, kelp, kombu, wakame, or dulse from sustainable sources. They are rich, salty, and earthy.

Strawberries

Strawberries' high vitamin C content aids in the production of collagen, which helps keep skin supple. Other constituents in these berries have been shown to kill certain cancer cells while helping normal cells repair themselves. They taste sweet and tart.

Sweet Potatoes

These root vegetables are high in omega-3 essential fatty acids to tonify the internal organs and strengthen immunity. They are rich in fiber for smooth transit time in the digestive system. Sweet potatoes come in a variety of colors: orange, purple, and white. The purple and white varieties are starchier and delicious when baked in breads. All purple produce contains anthocyanins, phytonutrients that are chemoprotective. Sweet potatoes are earthy, grounding, and sweet.

Winter Squash

Squashes are technically hearty fruits. They are rich in carotenoids, plant compounds that are antioxidant and anti-inflammatory. They contain vitamin A to support immunity and high potassium levels to promote muscle relaxation and bone density. Winter squash is high in manganese, which can help balance reproductive hormones and reduce premenstrual symptoms. Manganese and potassium together can help slow the process of lipogenesis, or fat production, and help the body use food for energy production instead of storage. Winter squash is sweet, light, and grounding.

WHOLE GRAINS

Amaranth

For Aztec people, amaranth is both a dietary staple and an important aspect of spiritual practice. It is an especially high-quality source of plant protein, including two essential amino acids, lysine and methionine, that are generally low in grains. Amaranth is gluten-free and easily digestible. It is antifungal and helps the body eliminate excess candida yeast. You can eat the greens as well as the seeds. Amaranth is primarily bitter in flavor.

Barley

This glutinous grain is an excellent source of insoluble fiber, thus creating less of a glycemic impact when digested. It contains eight essential amino acids to lend the body lasting nutrition. Barley is high in lignans, antioxidants that help reduce inflammation in the body. It is to be avoided by those with gluten sensitivity. Barley is unctuous, sweet, and slightly pungent.

Buckwheat

This little seed is not actually a grain but is often treated like one. It is gluten-free and contains more protein than fiber or fat. It is filling and nourishing, and it offers a warming quality that is welcome during the colder months. Buckwheat helps maintain balanced cholesterol, stable blood sugar, and low blood pressure. Its beneficial effects are due to its high flavonoid and magnesium content. It is earthy, nutty, and salty.

Corn

Although technically a vegetable, corn is considered a grain because it contains amylose starch, which maximizes its antioxidant value even when it's dried or ground into flour. It is high in fiber and B vitamins to promote digestion and maintain balanced blood glucose. The body accesses corn's vitamins and minerals most easily when corn has been nixtamalized, or treated with lime or wood ash. The word *nixtamal* comes from the Nahuatl *nixtli,* "ashes," and *tamalli,* "cooked corn." Aztec people discovered centuries ago that placing corn in a bath of water and wood ash or limestone powder made the kernels softer and easier to grind into masa, or corn flour. The nixtamal process makes two key nutrients in corn bioavailable to the human body: calcium and niacin. It tastes bittersweet.

Millet
Called the "queen of grains" in Chinese medicine, millet is neutral in nature, neither warming nor cooling but balancing to all constitutions. It is a nutrient-dense, hypoallergenic complex carbohydrate, and it offers a balance of B vitamins to support digestion and provide consistent energy. Those with thyroid challenges would do best to minimize millet. Millet tastes bitter and sweet.

Oats
High in fiber to lower cholesterol levels and reduce risk of heart disease, oats are grain of the grass family. They ease digestive stress and support healthy transit time. Oats enhance the immune response to infection and stabilize blood glucose. They calm and soothe the nervous system; oat straw or milky oat tea is commonly given to reduce stress in the European herbal tradition. Oats are sweet, soothing, and creamy.

Quinoa
This nutrient-dense complex carbohydrate offers a balance of B vitamins and magnesium to support digestion. It is useful in countering the mucus-forming effects of bread/cereal. High in essential amino acids for sustained energy, quinoa is a traditional food for Andean people who live at high altitudes. It is primarily bitter in flavor.

Rice

This member of the grass family is the most common cereal grain worldwide. It is nourishing and soothing to a system that's depleted, such as by cold or flu. It stops diarrhea, replenishes tissues, and is one of the easiest grains to digest. Rice that is unhulled (e.g., brown rice) maintains its bran and germ, the fiber and protein that the body needs to properly digest it. It contains phenolics, antioxidants that protect the body's tissues in the face of chronic stress and aging. Rice is sweet and creamy.

Rye

This grass family grain contains impressive amounts of manganese to maintain healthy bones, as well as insulinotropic polypeptides, plant chemicals that enhance body's insulin secretions for better digestion and absorption of this complex carbohydrate. Rye does contain gluten but expresses its proteins differently so that it is not as inflammatory as the gliadin protein found in wheat. It is sweet, earthy, and slightly sour.

PROTEINS

Beans

Rich in plant-based protein, these legumes provide readily available energy for the body to burn while maintaining balanced blood glucose with their high fiber content. Beans are rich in minerals and vitamins such as potassium, zinc, and folate. They are high in the amino acid lysine, which is beneficial for most but irritating to those who experience HSV1 (herpes). To gain a complete amino acid profile, match beans with rice; this simple and nourishing meal is consumed by cultures throughout the world. Beans taste sweet, earthy, and salty.

Beef

Grass-fed beef is rich in amino acids for energy and muscle strength. It is high in conjugated linoleic acid (CLA) to support balanced weight and a strong cardiovascular system. It can help balance blood glucose with its protein and saturated fat content and contains some omega-3 fatty acids due to the grasses that pastured cows eat. It also is high in niacin and zinc to promote stress relief and immunity. Beef is sweet, sour, and earthy.

Chicken

Chicken provides a balance of fats and amino acids for energy production, gut healing, and glandular support. The amino acids in chicken specifically help support the thyroid and adrenal glands. It also contains collagen as well as vitamins A and D for bone health, gut lining repair, and immune support. Try to purchase pastured chicken so that you gain the nutrients that are transferred to the meat when chickens eat grubs, worms, and other insects. Chicken is slightly sweet as well as sour and rich.

Eggs

Each egg contains approximately 6 grams of protein, nine essential amino acids, and 1.5 grams of saturated fat. Eggs are rich in lutein, which helps prevent macular degeneration and cataracts. They help maintain healthy cholesterol balance and are a source of vitamin D. Eggs are also high in choline, the precursor chemical for acetylcholine, one of the body's most fundamental neurotransmitters and hormone regulators. Try to eat eggs from pastured chickens to gain their fatty acid benefit. Only chickens that forage in the fields where they can consume grasses and insects are able to convert those nutrients into omega-3 and omega-6 fatty acids. Eggs have a rich, salty flavor.

Fish

Fish contains beneficial fats and amino acids, naturally occurring vitamin D, and lutein, which helps prevent macular degeneration and cataracts. It also helps to balance overall cholesterol. Fatty fish such as salmon, sardines, mackerel, anchovies, and herring are the best choice for gaining anti-inflammatory EPA and DHA fatty acids. Fish is salty, unctuous, and a bit bitter.

SWEETENERS

Honey

Antibacterial, antiviral, and antifungal, honey supports a healthy respiratory system and proliferation of beneficial gut bacteria. It is vulnerary and can be applied to burns and cuts to expedite healing. Mix it with minced garlic and eat a few tablespoons daily for a potent cold remedy. Local, raw honey may help the body respond better to pollen allergies. Honey is comprised entirely of fructose, a sugar that can be difficult to digest for those with harmful bacterial overgrowth in the small intestine. It is both sweet and bitter.

Maple Syrup

Maple syrup is rich in beneficial probiotic bacteria as well as prebiotic compounds to help feed those bacteria. It is lower on the glycemic index than refined beet/cane sugar and honey, so it doesn't impact blood glucose as much as other sweeteners. It's high in magnesium for muscle relaxation and niacin for brain health. Its polyphenol antioxidants help reduce inflammation, especially in the case of gut-related disorders such as irritable bowel syndrome (IBS). It is both sweet and a bit sour.

HERBS AND SPICES

Allspice

The allspice berry is highly antimicrobial and important for those who live in climates where parasitic and fungal infections are common. It supports balanced blood pressure by promoting circulation and helps heal conditions such as gout by lowering inflammation. The analgesic (pain-relieving) aspect of this spice makes it helpful in tooth or gum infections. Allspice is rich, complex, sweet, bitter, slightly sour, and pungent.

Basil

This herb is antibacterial, antispasmodic, digestive, tonic, and aromatic. It contains water-soluble flavonoids that stimulate the growth of white blood cells and protect cells from radiation and oxidative stress. Its volatile essential oils help balance gut flora. Basil is bitter and cooling.

Cardamom

This fragrant seed contains a phytochemical that helps break down digestive mucus, thus reducing gas and bloating, primarily from dairy products. It freshens the breath, brings sweetness to unsweetened desserts, and is slightly cooling. Cardamom is bitter and aromatic.

Cilantro

The leaf of this plant has been cultivated and used as a culinary herb in cultures from India to Europe for centuries. The seed, coriander, has similar effects to cilantro. This phytonutrient-rich herb stimulates the secretion of insulin and helps lower levels of total cholesterol, while increasing levels of HDL cholesterol. Cilantro and coriander's volatile oils have antimicrobial properties and taste both bitter and sweet. Cilantro is more cooling and coriander more warming.

Cinnamon

The ground version of this bark stimulates the pancreas to produce digestive enzymes and also makes the body more receptive to insulin, thus balancing blood sugar and reducing triglycerides. It contains phytonutrients that reduce pain and inflammation. Its antimicrobial activity helps ward off the cold and flu and reduce the overgrowth of *Candida albicans* yeast in the gut. Cinnamon is sweet, warming, and slightly pungent.

Ginger

Ginger is anti-inflammatory, soothes stomach cramps, reduces flatulence, and alleviates common cold and flu symptoms. Clinical studies show that ginger consumption decreases arthritis pain and protects the liver from damage. It is warming, pungent, and slightly sweet.

Nutmeg

This complex and fragrant seed is high in manganese for strong bones and healthy immune response. Its high volatile oil content makes it antifungal, anti-inflammatory, carminative, stomachic, and hypolipidemic. It is incredibly supportive to balanced digestion. Nutmeg tastes rich, sweet, and slightly pungent.

Parsley

In small doses, this potent perennial herb helps cleanse the kidneys and gallbladder. It is rich in vitamin C to decrease inflammation, beta-carotene to help prevent infection and strengthen immunity, and folic acid to support cardiovascular health. It contains volatile oils that can help neutralize particular types of carcinogens as well as ease the burn of insect bites and stings. Choose flat-leaf varieties (as opposed to curly), which contain more minerals. It is bitter and balancing.

Peppermint

As a cooling stomachic, peppermint relieves indigestion, dyspepsia, and colonic muscle spasms by relaxing the smooth muscle tissue of the intestines. Peppermint contains rosmarinic acid, which helps open bronchial passageways and reduce the effects of allergy-induced cold symptoms. It also has abundant phytochemicals that inhibit the formation of coronary plaques, and it helps combat *Helicobacter pylori* bacteria, whose overgrowth can cause stomach ulcers. Peppermint is cooling, sweet, bitter, and drying.

Rosemary

This antiseptic herb contains rosmarinic acid, which stimulates the immune system, increases circulation, and improves digestion and concentration. Anti-inflammatory, digestive, and aromatic, rosemary both aids in digesting fats and decreases the risk of infection from contaminated foods. Rosemary is warming, sour, bitter, and moist.

Sage

Sage improves memory by decreasing the growth of neurovascular plaque in the brain. It soothes the digestive tract, dries excess mucus from all membranes, and provides crucial phytonutrients that counteract the effects of oxidation, not only in human blood but also in cooking oils and nuts. It can be used to dry up breast milk supply in lactating bodies. Sage is warming, dry, bitter, and astringent.

Thyme

Thyme contains thymol and other volatile oils that have antimicrobial activity against bacteria, thereby helping to preserve foods and protect them from microbial contamination. Thymol helps increase the percentage of healthy fats, such as DHA, in brain, kidney, and heart cell membranes. Thyme is warming, sweet, and bitter.

Tulsi

Sweet, floral, and spicy, tulsi (sometimes called holy basil) has been used for thousands of years in Ayurveda for its diverse healing properties. It is an adaptogen, helpful for adapting to stress. Marked by its strong aroma and astringent taste, it is believed to promote longevity. Extracts made from the leaves and flowers of this plant are used for headaches, stomach disorders, inflammation, blood sugar imbalances, and the common cold. A member of the mint family, tulsi is cooling, bitter, and sweet.

Turmeric

Turmeric contains anti-inflammatory curcumin, which helps heal gastrointestinal diseases such as irritable bowel syndrome. It prevents cancer cells from growing new blood vessels to feed themselves and induces the death of existing cancer cells. It also breaks up accumulated amyloid plaque in the brain that's related to the onset of Alzheimer's disease. Turmeric is warming and bitter.

This list represents a beginning. You can begin to create your own culinary pharmacy as you notice which foods intuitively call to you and learn the reason why you benefit from them. One of my favorite books is *The Whole Foods Encyclopedia* by Rebecca Wood. It contains many more foods (but not animal foods) and more details about each one. The ChineseNutrition.org website offers a wealth of information about most any food you could imagine as well as each food's organ association, flavors, and thermal nature. You can start to compile your list of healing foods, as well as ones that challenge you, based on this information and your intuition about a food's specific actions in your physical, mental, and spiritual bodies.

What is your purpose in this lifetime? What did you come here in this human form to offer? How can you heal yourself so that you can contribute to the healing of the planet? Food is the foundation for restoring connection between self, nature, and the unseen world that animates all things. Emotions lead to thoughts; thoughts create words; words create reality. The reality of life is sacred and ever changing. We live in a world that is at once hopeful and fraught with fear of the unknown. Hope and fear are two sides of the same coin. When we touch them both, we know that integration and true healing are possible. When we use food as a tool to align with who we are, beyond cravings, addictions, patterns, or mindless habits, we can begin to glimpse the spiritual reality taught in traditional healing systems worldwide. May all beings be safe. May all beings be well. May all beings know peace.

Notes

I. THE ROOTS OF FOOD AS MEDICINE

1. Frank W. Stahnisch and Marja Verhoef, "The Flexner Report of 1910 and Its Impact on Complementary and Alternative Medicine and Psychiatry in North America in the 20th Century," *Evidence-Based Complementary Alternative Medicine,* December 26, 2012.

2. CONSTITUTION INFORMS NOURISHMENT

1. Zhang Yifang and Yao Yingzhi, *Your Guide to Health with Foods and Herbs* (Shanghai Press, 2012), 57.
2. Five Seasons TCM, "The Nine Body Constitutions," online post, accessed June 1, 2022.
3. Worts and Cunning Apothecary, "The Four Elements of Traditional Western Herbalism," online post, last modified August 9, 2021.
4. Casey Seidenberg, "Kombu, A Nutritional Powerhouse from the Sea," The Washington Post (website), January 29, 2013.
5. Sara Al-Rawi, "Traditional Arabic and Islamic Medicine," *Global Journal of Health Sciences,* May 2012, 164–69.
6. Renaldo Maduro, "Curanderismo and Latino Views of Disease and Curing," *Western Journal of Medicine,* December 1983, 868–74.

3. ORGANS, SEASONS, AND SYSTEMS

1. Bill Mollison, *Permaculture: A Designer's Manual* (Tagari Publications, 1998).

2. Land Institute, "The Land Institute," website home page, accessed July 1, 2022.

4. TOWARD INTUITIVE EATING

1. Quoted in Sandee LaMotte, "Intuitive Eating: The Anti-Diet, or How Pleasure from Food Is the Answer, Say Its Creators," CNN (website), January 31, 2020.
2. Dariush Mozaffarian, "Perspective: Obesity—An Unexplained Epidemic," *American Journal of Clinical Nutrition,* June 2022, 1445–50, doi. org/10.1093/ajcn/nqac075.
3. SUSU CommUNITY Farm, "Unbodying White Bodied Supremacy," online post, accessed August 1, 2022.
4. Cristine H. Legare and André L. Souza, "Evaluating Ritual Efficacy: Evidence from the Supernatural," *Cognition,* July 2012, 124.

5. TRUSTING YOUR GUT

1. Tina Hesman Saey, "Gut Bacteria Come in Three Flavors," *Science News,* April 20, 2011.
2. Manimozhiyan Arumugam, Jeroen Raes, Eric Pelletier, Denis Le Paslier, Takuji Yamada, Daniel R. Mende, Peer Bork, et al., "Enterotypes of the Human Gut Microbiome," *Nature,* April 20, 2011, 473.
3. Emily R. Davenport, Orna Mizrahi-Man, Katelyn Michelini, Luis B. Barreiro, Carole Ober, and Gilad Yoav, "Seasonal Variation in Human Gut Microbiome Composition," *Plos One,* March 11, 2014.
4. M. Nathaniel Mead, "Nutrigenomics: The Genome–Food Interface," *Environmental Health Perspectives,* December 2007, 115.
5. Nobuyuki Sudo et al., "Postnatal Microbial Colonization Programs the Hypothalamic-Pituitary-Adrenal System for Stress Response in Mice," *Journal of Physiology* 558, pt. 1 (2004): 263–75.
6. Bruno Bonaz, Thomas Bazin, and Sonia Pellissier, "The Vagus Nerve at the Interface of the Microbiota-Gut-Brain Axis," *Frontiers in Neuroscience,* February 7, 2018.
7. Bethany E. Kok, Kimberly A. Coffey, Michael A. Cohn, Lahnna I. Catalino, Tanya Vacharkulksemsuk, Sara B. Algoe, Mary Brantley, and Barbara L. Fredrickson, "How Positive Emotions Build Physical Health:

Perceived Positive Social Connections Account for the Upward Spiral between Positive Emotions and Vagal Tone," *Psychological Science,* July 1, 2013.

8. S. E. Erdman and T. Poutahidis, "Probiotic 'Glow of Health': It's More than Skin Deep," *Beneficial Microbes,* June 2014, 109–19.

9. Julio Plaza-Diaz, Francisco Javier Ruiz-Ojeda, Mercedes Gil-Campos, and Angel Gil, "Mechanisms of Action of Probiotics," *Advanced Nutrition,* February 9, 2019, S49–66.

10. Rasu Jayabalan, V. Radomir, Eva Malbaša, Jasmina Lončar, S. Vitas, and Sathishkumar Muthuswamy, "A Review on Kombucha Tea—Microbiology, Composition, Fermentation, Beneficial Effects, Toxicity, and Tea Fungus," *Comprehensive Reviews in Food Science and Food Safety,* June 2014.

11. Daiara Tukano, "The First Indigenous Ayahuasca Conference (Yubaka Hayrá) in Acre Demonstrates Political, Cultural and Spiritual Resistance," Chacruna, Institute for Psychedelic Plant Medicines (website), February 2019.

6. NUTRIENTS AND WELLNESS

1. J. G. Salway, *Metabolism at a Glance,* 2nd ed. (Blackwell Science, 1999).

2. Jaime Vengoechea and Kent D. McKelvey, "Cholesterol and Family History: When Genetics Matters," *Journal of the Arkansas Medical Society,* February 2015.

3. Seyede-Masome Derakhshande-Rishehri, Marjan Mansourian, Roya Kelishadi, and Motahar Heidari-Beni, "Association of Foods Enriched in Conjugated Linoleic Acid (CLA) and CLA Supplements with Lipid Profile in Human Studies: A Systematic Review and Meta-analysis," *Public Health Nutrition,* August 2015.

4. The Vegan Society, "Definition of Veganism," Website, accessed April 26, 2023.

7. PERSONALIZED NUTRITION PLANS

1. Herman Pontzer, Yosuke Yamada, Hiroyuki Sagayama, Philip N. Ainslie, Lene F. Anderse, Liam J. Anderson, Lenore Arab, Issadd Baddou, et al., "Daily Energy Expenditure through the Human Life Course," *Science,* August 2021, 808–12.

2. Mark P. Mattson, Tae Gen Son, and Simonetta Camandola, "Viewpoint: Mechanisms of Action and Therapeutic Potential of Neurohormetic Phytochemicals," *Dose Response,* August 2007, 174–86.

9. FOOD SOVEREIGNTY

1. Susy Ferrazde Oliveira, Ivon Pinheiro Lôbo, Rosenira Serpada da Cruz, João Luciano Andriolia, et al., "Antimicrobial Activity of Coconut Oil-in-Water Emulsion on *Staphylococcus epidermidis* and *Escherichia coli,*" *Heliyon,* November 2018, doi.org/10.1016/j.heliyon.2018.e00924.
2. Food and Agriculture Organization of the United Nations, "The State of Food Security and Nutrition in the World 2021," Website, accessed April 26, 2023.
3. Food and Agriculture Organization of the United Nations, "The State of Food Security and Nutrition in the World 2021," Website, accessed April 26, 2023.
4. Ana Moragues-Faus, "Distributive Food Systems to Build Just and Liveable Futures," *Agriculture and Human Values* 37, no. 3 (2020): 583–84.

Bibliography

Abraham, Ellen. *Simple Treats.* Summertown, TN: Book Publishing Company, 1972.

Alford, Jefferey, and Naomi Duguid. *Flatbreads and Flavors.* New York: William Morrow, 2008.

Balch, Phyllis A. *Prescription for Nutritional Healing.* New York: Avery Publishing Group, 2007.

Brown, Edward Espe. *No Recipe: Cooking as a Spiritual Practice.* Louisville, CO: Sounds True, 2018.

Colbin, Annemarie. *Food and Healing.* New York: Random House, 1986.

Cunningham, Marion. *The Breakfast Book.* New York: Random House, 1987.

Fallon, Sally. *Nourishing Traditions.* White Plains, MD: New Trends Publishing, 1992.

Flexner, Abraham. *Medical Education in the United States and Canada: A Report to the Carnegie Foundation for the Advancement of Teaching.* New York: Carnegie Foundation for the Advancement of Teaching, 1910.

Fogg, B. J. *Tiny Habits.* New York: HarperCollins, 2019.

Hanh, Thich Nhat, and Dr. Lillian Cheung. *Savor: Mindful Eating, Mindful Life.* New York: HarperCollins, 2011.

Hof, Wim. *The Wim Hof Method: Activate Your Full Human Potential.* Louisville, CO: Sounds True, 2020.

Kaptchuk, Ted. *The Web That Has No Weaver: Understanding Chinese Medicine.* New York: McGraw Hill, 2000.

Katz, Sandor Ellix. *The Art of Fermentation.* White River Junction, VT: Chelsea Green, 2012.

Linus Pauling Institute. "Micronutrient Information Center." Linus Pauling Institute at Oregon State University (online). Accessed June 1, 2022.

Mateljan, George. *The World's Healthiest Foods: Essential Guide for the Healthiest Way of Eating*. George Mateljan Foundation, 2006.

Mintz, Sydney. *Sweetness and Power*. New York: Penguin Books, 1986.

Mueller, Tom. *Extra Virginity: The Sublime and Scandalous World of Olive Oil*. New York: W. W. Norton and Company, 2013.

Murray, Michael T., and Joseph Pizzorno. *The Encyclopedia of Healing Foods*. Lousville, KY: Atria, 2005.

Murray, Michael T., and Joseph Pizzorno. *The Encyclopedia of Natural Medicine*, third edition. Lousville, KY: Atria, 2012.

Nestor, James. *Breath: The New Science of a Lost Art*. New York: Riverhead Books, 2020.

Ni, Maoshing. *The Yellow Emperor's Classic of Medicine: A New Translation of the Neijing Suwen with Commentary*. Boulder, CO: Shambhala, 1995.

Nosrat, Samin. *Salt, Fat, Acid, Heat: Mastering the Elements of Good Cooking*. New York: Simon & Schuster, 2017.

Onstad, Dianne. *Whole Foods Companion*. White River Junction, VT: Chelsea Green, 2004.

Patel, Raj. *Stuffed and Starved: The Hidden Battle for the World Food System*. New York: Melville House, 2012.

Pieroni, Andrea, and Lisa Leimer Price. *Eating and Healing: Traditional Food as Medicine*. Boca Raton, FL: CRC Press, 2006.

Pisharodi, Sanjay. *Acharya Vagbhata's Astanga Hrdayam*, volume 1 of *The Essence of Ayurveda*. Uttar Pradesh, India: Purnarogya Holistic Healing Centre, 2016.

Pitchford, Paul. *Healing with Whole Foods*. Berkeley, CA: North Atlantic Books, 1993.

Pollan, Michael. *In Defense of Food: An Eater's Manifesto*. New York: Penguin Books, 2009.

Pontzer, Herman. *Burn: New Research Blows the Lid Off How We Really Burn Calories, Lose Weight, and Stay Healthy*. New York: Avery, 2021.

Prentice, Jessica. *Full Moon Feast*. White River Junction, VT: Chelsea Green, 2007.

Segnit, Nikki. *The Flavor Thesaurus*. London: Bloomsbury, 2010.

Taylor, Sonya Renee. *The Body Is Not an Apology: The Power of Radical Self-Love*. Oakland, CA: Berrett-Koehler Publishers, 2018.

Tiwari, Maya. *Ayurveda: A Life of Balance*. Rochester, VT: Healing Arts Press, 1993.

Tribole, Evelyn and Elyse Resch. *Intuitive Eating,* fourth edition. New York: St. Martin's Press, 2020.

Turner, Kristina. *The Self-Healing Cookbook.* Vashon, WA: Earthtones Press, 1996.

Walters, Terry. *Clean Food.* New York: Sterling Epicure, 2009.

Wood, Rebecca. *The New Whole Foods Encyclopedia.* New York: Penguin, 2010.

Yifang, Zhang, and Yao Yingzhi. *Your Guide to Health with Foods and Herbs.* Shanghai, China: Shanghai Press, 2012.

Index

Page numbers in *italics* refer to illustrations